30 minutes solution parkinson disease diet Cookbook: for seniors

Fast and easy complete delicious 100+recipes to deactivate seniors pain, with special 28day meal plan to balance seniors healthy.

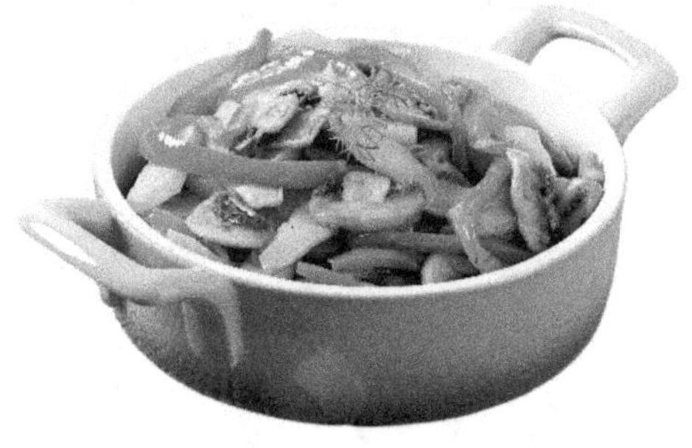

Dr. Jerry Cole

TABLE OF CONTENT

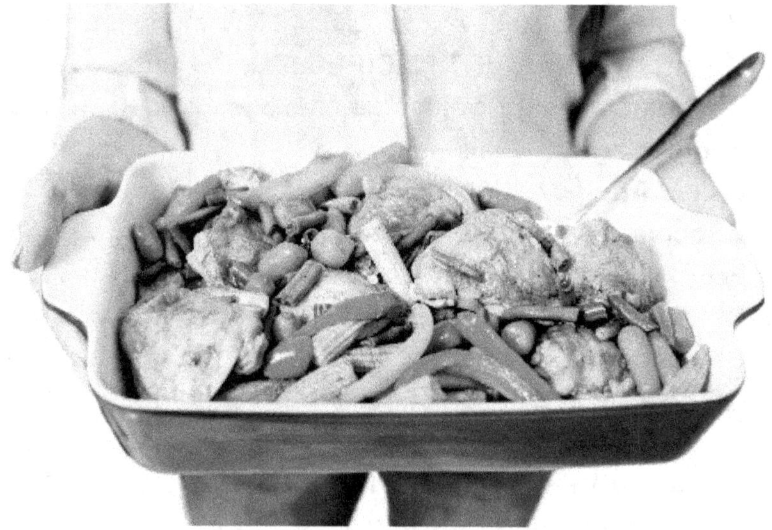

INTRODUCTION

"Welcome to the 30-Minute Solution Parkinson's Disease Diet Cookbook for Seniors!

As we age, our bodies undergo many changes, and managing Parkinson's disease can become an added challenge. But what if you could take control of your nutrition and cook delicious, healthy meals in just 30 minutes or less?

This cookbook is designed specifically for seniors living with Parkinson's disease, with easy-to-follow recipes and simple ingredients to make cooking a breeze. Our goal is to empower you to take charge of your diet and nutrition, and to make a positive impact on your overall health and well-being.

Inside these pages, you'll find:

- 100+ quick and easy recipes tailored to Parkinson's disease dietary needs

- Nutritious and wholesome ingredients to support brain health and overall well-being
- Step-by-step instructions and photos to make cooking a breeze
- Tips and tricks for meal prep, cooking, and nutrition

Cooking doesn't have to be a chore - it can be a joyful experience that brings people together and nourishes our bodies and souls. So let's get cooking, and start enjoying the benefits of a healthy Parkinson's disease diet today!"

This introduction aims to:

- Welcome and reassure the reader
- Emphasize the importance of nutrition in managing Parkinson's disease
- Introduce the cookbook and its benefits
- Preview the content and features of the cookbook
- Encourage the reader to start cooking and taking control of their health

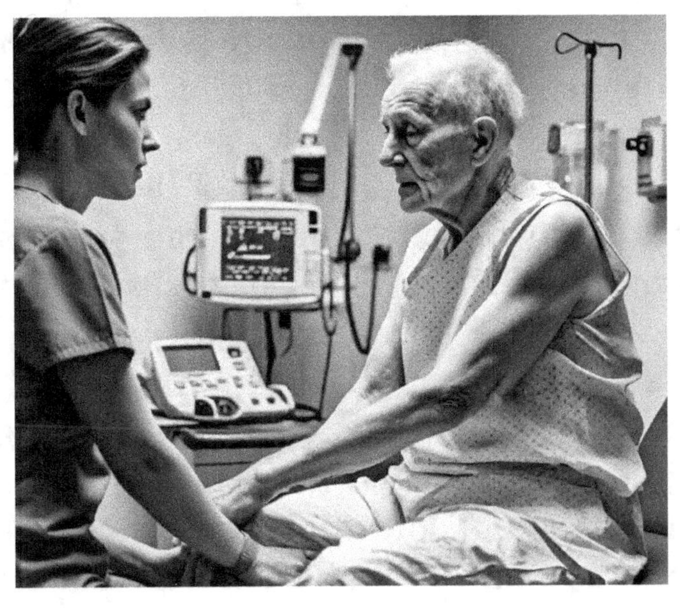

One neurodegenerative condition that mostly impairs movement is Parkinson's disease. It usually begins slowly, with a minor tremor in one hand, and then spreads to other regions of the body. Tremors, bradykinesia (slowed movement), rigidity (stiffness of the limbs and trunk), and poor balance and coordination are the prominent symptoms.

The substantia nigra, a part of the brain, is where dopamine-producing brain cells are lost, and this is what causes Parkinson's disease. One neurotransmitter that is essential for controlling movement and emotional reactions is dopamine. Although the precise etiology of Parkinson's disease cell loss is unknown, it most likely results from a confluence of environmental and hereditary variables.

Parkinson's disease cannot be cured, however there are therapies to assist control its symptoms. Medication, physical therapy, occupational therapy, and even surgery in more severe situations are some of these treatments.

Chapter 2:DIETARY REQUIREMENTS FOR ELDERS WITH PARKINSON'S DISEASE

Seniors with Parkinson's disease should eat a nutritious, well-balanced diet to assist control their symptoms and preserve general health. The following food guidelines should be followed by those who have Parkinson's disease:

High-Fiber Foods: Parkinson's disease patients frequently have constipation as a result of their sluggish digestion. Constipation can be lessened by eating foods high in fiber, such as fruits, vegetables, whole grains, and legumes.

Protein Management: It's crucial to distribute your protein intake throughout the day rather than ingesting a lot at once because some Parkinson's treatments can make it difficult for your body to absorb protein. Lean meats, poultry, fish, eggs, dairy products, tofu, and legumes are all excellent sources of protein.

Foods High in Antioxidants: Antioxidants may help prevent damage to brain cells. Add in lots of fruits and vegetables, particularly those high in antioxidants (such vitamins C and E) including kale, spinach, berries, and citrus fruits.

Omega-3 Fatty Acids: Foods high in omega-3 fatty acids, such walnuts, flaxseeds, chia seeds, and fatty fish (salmon, mackerel, and sardines), may have anti-inflammatory qualities that help people with Parkinson's disease.

Hydration: Symptoms like constipation and urinary tract infections might get worse if you're dehydrated. Promote a sufficient intake of fluids, mainly from water, herbal teas, and meals that are high in water content, such as soups and fruits.

Vitamin D: This nutrient is necessary for healthy bones, muscles, and maybe even the nervous system. Seniors with Parkinson's disease should make sure they get enough vitamin D from meals like cereals and dairy products that have been fortified, as well as from sunshine when they can.

Little, Regular Meals: Smaller, more frequent meals spread out throughout the day can aid in the management of digestive problems and help avoid Parkinson's disease-related weariness.

Avoiding Specific Foods: Certain foods and beverages, such as alcohol, caffeine, and high-fat foods, may make symptoms worse for some people with Parkinson's disease. Observe the effects of various foods on symptoms and modify the diet accordingly.

Individualized Nutrition Plan: It's critical for people to collaborate with a healthcare professional or registered dietitian to create a personalized nutrition plan that suits their unique requirements and preferences, as Parkinson's disease symptoms and progression can differ greatly from person to person.

Seniors with Parkinson's disease can benefit from a balanced diet that is high in fruits, vegetables, whole grains, lean protein, and healthy fats as it can promote general health and wellbeing.

In order to help elders manage Parkinson's disease and preserve their quality of life, there are a few essential steps that need to be taken at the outset. Here's a how-to for getting going:

Medical Assessment: Make an appointment for a comprehensive assessment and diagnosis of Parkinson's disease with a healthcare professional, ideally a neurologist or movement disorder expert. The results of this evaluation will inform therapy choices and assist ascertain the severity of the ailment.

drug Management: Talk to the healthcare professional about your drug options. Levodopa, dopamine agonists, and MAO-B inhibitors are among the drugs that are frequently used to treat Parkinson's symptoms. Comprehending the dosage, possible adverse effects, and appropriate time of medicine administration is crucial.

Exercise Routine: Encourage them to engage in a regular fitness regimen that suits their interests and skills. Exercise has been demonstrated to enhance a person with Parkinson's disease's movement, balance, and general well-being. Exercises like cycling, tai chi, yoga, swimming, and walking can be advantageous.

Physical Therapy: You might want to think about signing up for a program that is especially tailored for people with Parkinson's disease. In addition to treating gait and balance problems, physical therapists can offer exercises and strategies to enhance strength, flexibility, posture, and mobility.

Speech Therapy: Speech therapy is a useful tool for seniors with Parkinson's disease to preserve or enhance their ability to swallow, project their voice, and communicate. speaking therapists can provide exercises and techniques to help with swallowing and speaking issues.

Occupational Therapy: To preserve their independence and safety, seniors with Parkinson's disease can modify their everyday activities and routines with the help of occupational therapists. They can offer advice on home adaptations, assistive technology, and methods for handling daily living activities.

Nutritional Support: Consult a certified dietitian to create a well-balanced and nutrient-dense meal plan that takes into account any unique dietary requirements or issues associated with Parkinson's disease, such as managing protein intake, staying hydrated, and preventing constipation.

Support Groups: Promote involvement in nearby support groups or virtual communities catering to Parkinson's disease patients and their carers. Making connections with people going through comparable struggles can offer a feeling of community, helpful guidance, and emotional support.

Support for Caregivers: In the event that a caregiver is involved, make sure they have access to tools and services that will assist them in handling the duties and difficulties associated with providing care. This could involve counseling, education about Parkinson's illness, and respite care.

Frequent Follow-Up: Make follow-up appointments on a frequent basis with your healthcare provider to track the advancement of Parkinson's disease, make any medication adjustments, and discuss any new symptoms or concerns.

Seniors with Parkinson's disease can effectively manage their condition and preserve their independence and quality of life for as long as feasible by taking these first actions and obtaining the necessary help and resources.

Cooking together with elderly people who have Parkinson's disease can be a fulfilling and pleasurable experience, but it might need to be modified to meet their unique requirements and limitations. Here are some pointers for elders with Parkinson's disease while they cook:

Make a plan in advance and select recipes that are easy to follow and have minimal ingredients. To reduce the amount of chopping, slicing, and other fine motor skill-demanding tasks, think about prepping materials.

Use Adaptive Equipment: Seniors with Parkinson's disease can cook more safely and more easily by using adapted kitchen tools and utensils. Jar openers, non-slip cutting boards, and ergonomic cutlery with bigger handles are a few examples of useful items.

Establish a secure cooking space: Make sure there are no trip hazards in the kitchen, such as loose rugs or clutter, and that it is well-lit. To reduce the amount of bending or straining required, place kitchen tools and ingredients in an accessible location.

Promote Involvement: As far as possible, involve elders in the culinary process while keeping in mind their limitations and skills. Assign them jobs like stirring, pouring, or assembling components that they can perform with ease.

Support: Assist and advise as required, but let elders keep their freedom and self-sufficiency in the kitchen. Show them your patience and support while praising and encouraging their efforts.

Techniques should be modified to account for any physical restrictions or tremors brought on by Parkinson's disease. For instance, chop and puree using a food processor or blender, and whenever possible, utilize pre-cut fruits and vegetables.

Keep an eye on cooking times and heat: To avoid burns or overcooking, pay great attention to the stovetop temperature and cooking periods. When cooking dishes that call for simmering or braising, think about utilizing lower heat settings and longer cooking times.

Make Cleaning Easy: Utilize disposable or easily cleaned cookware and utensils to reduce mess and cleanup. Seniors should be urged to tidy their cooking area by cleaning as they go.

Put Pleasure First: Place more of an emphasis on having fun while preparing and serving meals than on attaining culinary perfection. In the kitchen, promote experimentation and innovation, and value the steps involved just as much as the product.

Remain Adaptable: Be ready to modify your strategy in response to the particular requirements and tastes of the senior you're cooking for. As each individual with

Parkinson's disease is different, cook with flexibility and consideration for others.

Cooking together can be an amazing method to boost cognitive function, engage senses, and foster social contact and connection for elders with Parkinson's disease. You can make cooking together a meaningful and enjoyable hobby for the two of you if you have patience, creativity, and a focus on safety and enjoyment.

Chapter 5:28DAY MEAL PLAN

Day 1:

- Breakfast: Oatmeal topped with sliced bananas and chopped walnuts. Serve with a side of Greek yogurt.
- Lunch: Grilled salmon served with quinoa and steamed broccoli.
- Dinner: Baked chicken breast with roasted sweet potatoes and a spinach

salad with strawberries and balsamic vinaigrette.

Day 2:

- Breakfast: Whole grain toast topped with avocado and a poached egg. Serve with a side of mixed berries.
- Lunch: Turkey and avocado wrap made with whole grain tortilla, served with a side of vegetable soup.
- Dinner: Stir-fried tofu with mixed vegetables and brown rice. Serve with a side of steamed edamame.

Day 3:

- Breakfast: Smoothie made with spinach, kale, banana, almond milk, and a scoop of protein powder.
- Lunch: Lentil soup served with a side of whole grain crackers and a mixed green salad.

- Dinner: Grilled shrimp skewers with roasted vegetables (such as bell peppers, zucchini, and onions) and quinoa.

Day 4:

- Breakfast: Greek yogurt parfait layered with granola and mixed berries.
- Lunch: Chicken and vegetable stir-fry with brown rice.
- Dinner: Baked cod fillets with steamed asparagus and mashed sweet potatoes.

Day 5:

- Breakfast: Whole grain cereal with almond milk and sliced peaches.
- Lunch: Quinoa salad with diced vegetables, chickpeas, and a lemon-tahini dressing.
- Dinner: Turkey meatballs served with whole wheat spaghetti and marinara

sauce. Serve with a side of roasted Brussels sprouts.

Day 6:

- Breakfast: Whole grain pancakes topped with Greek yogurt and mixed berries.
- Lunch: Spinach and feta omelet served with whole grain toast and a side of fruit salad.
- Dinner: Beef and vegetable stew served with whole grain dinner rolls.

Day 7:

- Breakfast: Scrambled eggs with sautéed spinach and mushrooms. Serve with whole grain toast.
- Lunch: Grilled vegetable panini made with whole grain bread and served with a side of tomato soup.

- Dinner: Baked salmon with a lemon-dill sauce, roasted potatoes, and steamed green beans.

Day 8:

- Breakfast: Smoothie bowl topped with sliced bananas, berries, almonds, and a drizzle of honey.
- Lunch: Grilled chicken Caesar salad with romaine lettuce, grilled chicken breast, whole grain croutons, and a light Caesar dressing.
- Dinner: Baked tilapia with roasted root vegetables (carrots, parsnips, and beets) and a side of quinoa pilaf.

Day 9:

- Breakfast: Whole grain toast topped with almond butter and sliced apples. Serve with a side of cottage cheese.
- Lunch: Lentil and vegetable curry served with brown rice.

- Dinner: Turkey chili made with lean
  ground turkey, beans, tomatoes, and
  spices. Serve with a side of whole grain
  cornbread.

Day 10:

- Breakfast: Yogurt parfait with layers of
  Greek yogurt, granola, and mixed
  berries.
- Lunch: Grilled vegetable and hummus
  wrap made with whole grain tortilla.
  Serve with a side of carrot and celery
  sticks.
- Dinner: Baked chicken thighs with
  roasted Brussels sprouts and quinoa.

Day 11:

- Breakfast: Spinach and mushroom
  omelet served with whole grain toast
  and sliced oranges.

- Lunch: Quinoa and black bean salad with diced tomatoes, corn, avocado, and lime-cilantro dressing.
- Dinner: Beef and broccoli stir-fry served with brown rice.

Day 12:

- Breakfast: Whole grain cereal with sliced bananas and almond milk.
- Lunch: Mediterranean-style tuna salad made with canned tuna, olives, cherry tomatoes, cucumbers, and feta cheese. Serve with whole grain crackers.
- Dinner: Baked cod with roasted cauliflower and a mixed green salad.

Day 13:

- Breakfast: Whole grain waffles topped with Greek yogurt and mixed berries.

- Lunch: Turkey and vegetable soup served with a side of whole grain bread.
- Dinner: Grilled shrimp tacos with cabbage slaw and avocado salsa. Serve with a side of black beans.

Day 14:

- Breakfast: Smoothie made with spinach, mango, pineapple, Greek yogurt, and coconut water.
- Lunch: Chickpea and avocado salad with mixed greens, cherry tomatoes, and a lemon-tahini dressing.
- Dinner: Baked chicken drumsticks with roasted sweet potatoes and steamed green beans.

Day 15:

- Breakfast: Whole grain pancakes topped with sliced strawberries and a drizzle of honey. Serve with a side of Greek yogurt.

- Lunch: Grilled vegetable and quinoa salad with a lemon vinaigrette dressing.
- Dinner: Baked salmon with roasted asparagus and a side of wild rice pilaf.

Day 16:

- Breakfast: Scrambled eggs with diced tomatoes and spinach. Serve with whole grain toast.
- Lunch: Turkey and avocado wrap made with whole grain tortilla, served with a side of vegetable soup.
- Dinner: Lentil stew with carrots, celery, and onions served with a side of whole grain bread.

Day 17:

- Breakfast: Smoothie made with kale, banana, almond milk, and a scoop of protein powder.
- Lunch: Chicken and vegetable stir-fry with brown rice.
- Dinner: Baked tofu with roasted Brussels sprouts and quinoa.

Day 18:

- Breakfast: Overnight oats made with rolled oats, almond milk, chia seeds, and topped with mixed berries.
- Lunch: Greek salad with mixed greens, cucumber, tomatoes, olives, feta cheese, and a lemon-herb vinaigrette.
- Dinner: Turkey meatballs served with whole wheat spaghetti and marinara sauce. Serve with a side of steamed broccoli.

Day 19:

- Breakfast: Whole grain toast topped with mashed avocado and sliced hard-boiled eggs. Serve with a side of mixed fruit.
- Lunch: Lentil soup served with a side of whole grain crackers and a mixed green salad.
- Dinner: Grilled chicken breast with roasted sweet potatoes and sautéed spinach.

Day 20:

- Breakfast: Greek yogurt parfait layered with granola and mixed berries.
- Lunch: Quinoa salad with diced vegetables, chickpeas, and a balsamic vinaigrette dressing.
- Dinner: Baked cod fillets with steamed green beans and quinoa.

Day 21:

- Breakfast: Whole grain cereal with almond milk and sliced peaches.
- Lunch: Spinach and feta omelet served with whole grain toast and a side of fruit salad.
- Dinner: Beef and vegetable stir-fry with brown rice.

Day 22:

- Breakfast: Whole grain toast with almond butter and sliced bananas. Serve with a side of Greek yogurt.
- Lunch: Turkey and vegetable stir-fry with brown rice.
- Dinner: Baked salmon with roasted Brussels sprouts and quinoa.

Day 23:

- Breakfast: Smoothie made with spinach, mango, banana, Greek yogurt, and almond milk.
- Lunch: Lentil and vegetable curry served with brown rice.
- Dinner: Grilled chicken breast with roasted sweet potatoes and steamed broccoli.

Day 24:

- Breakfast: Whole grain pancakes topped with mixed berries and a drizzle of maple syrup. Serve with a side of cottage cheese.
- Lunch: Quinoa and black bean salad with diced tomatoes, avocado, and a lime-cilantro dressing.
- Dinner: Baked tofu with sautéed spinach and quinoa.

Day 25:

- Breakfast: Scrambled eggs with diced tomatoes, onions, and spinach. Serve with whole grain toast.
- Lunch: Greek salad with mixed greens, cucumber, tomatoes, olives, feta cheese, and a lemon-herb vinaigrette.
- Dinner: Turkey chili made with lean ground turkey, beans, tomatoes, and spices. Serve with a side of whole grain cornbread.

Day 26:

- Breakfast: Yogurt parfait with layers of Greek yogurt, granola, and mixed berries.
- Lunch: Grilled vegetable and hummus wrap made with whole grain tortilla. Serve with a side of carrot and celery sticks.

- Dinner: Baked cod with roasted cauliflower and a mixed green salad.

Day 27:

- Breakfast: Whole grain cereal with almond milk and sliced peaches.
- Lunch: Lentil soup served with a side of whole grain crackers and a mixed green salad.
- Dinner: Beef and broccoli stir-fry with brown rice.

Day 28:

- Breakfast: Whole grain waffles topped with Greek yogurt and sliced strawberries.
- Lunch: Turkey and avocado sandwich on whole grain bread with a side of vegetable soup.
- Dinner: Baked chicken thighs with roasted root vegetables (carrots, parsnips, and potatoes) and quinoa.

Banana Oatmeal Porridge:

- Ingredients:
    1. 1 ripe banana
    2. 1/2 cup rolled oats
    3. 1 cup milk (dairy or plant-based)
    4. 1 tablespoon honey or maple syrup (optional)
- Instructions:
    1. In a saucepan, mash the banana.
    2. Add rolled oats and milk to the saucepan and cook over medium heat.
    3. Stir frequently until the oats are soft and the mixture thickens (about 5-7 minutes).
    4. Sweeten with honey or maple syrup if desired. Serve warm.

Scrambled Egg and Spinach Wrap:

- Ingredients:
    1. 2 eggs
    2. 1 cup fresh spinach leaves, chopped
    3. 2 whole wheat tortillas
    4. Salt and pepper to taste
- Instructions:
    1. Crack the eggs into a bowl, season with salt and pepper, and whisk.
    2. In a non-stick skillet, scramble the eggs over medium heat until cooked.
    3. Add the chopped spinach to the skillet and cook until wilted.
    4. Warm the tortillas in the microwave or on a skillet.
    5. Divide the scrambled egg and spinach mixture between the tortillas. Roll up and serve.

Greek Yogurt Parfait:

- Ingredients:
    1. 1 cup Greek yogurt
    2. 1/2 cup granola
    3. 1/2 cup mixed berries (strawberries, blueberries, raspberries)
    4. 1 tablespoon honey
- Instructions:
    1. In a serving glass or bowl, layer Greek yogurt, granola, and mixed berries.
    2. Drizzle honey over the top.
    3. Repeat the layers if desired.
    4. Serve immediately.

Smoothie with Protein:

- Ingredients:
    1. 1 ripe banana
    2. 1/2 cup frozen mixed berries
    3. 1/2 cup spinach leaves

4. 1/2 cup Greek yogurt
5. 1/2 cup milk (dairy or plant-based)
6. 1 scoop protein powder (optional)

- Instructions:
  1. Place all ingredients in a blender.
  2. Blend until smooth and creamy.
  3. If the smoothie is too thick, add more milk to reach the desired consistency.
  4. Pour into a glass and enjoy.

Apple Cinnamon Quinoa Porridge:

- Ingredients:
  1. 1/2 cup quinoa, rinsed
  2. 1 cup water
  3. 1 apple, diced
  4. 1/2 teaspoon cinnamon

5. 1 tablespoon honey or maple syrup (optional)

- ○ Instructions:
    1. In a saucepan, combine quinoa, water, diced apple, and cinnamon.
    2. Bring to a boil, then reduce the heat and simmer until the quinoa is cooked and the liquid is absorbed (about 15-20 minutes).
    3. Stir in honey or maple syrup if desired.
    4. Serve warm.

Peanut Butter Banana Toast:

- ○ Ingredients:
    1. 2 slices whole wheat bread
    2. 2 tablespoons peanut butter
    3. 1 banana, sliced
    4. 1 teaspoon honey (optional)

- ○ Instructions:
    1. Toast the slices of whole wheat bread until golden brown.
    2. Spread peanut butter evenly on each slice.
    3. Arrange banana slices on top of the peanut butter.
    4. Drizzle with honey if desired. Serve immediately.

Vegetable Egg Muffins:

- ○ Ingredients:
    1. 4 eggs
    2. 1/4 cup milk (dairy or plant-based)
    3. 1/2 cup diced vegetables (bell peppers, spinach, onions, mushrooms, etc.)
    4. Salt and pepper to taste
- ○ Instructions:

1. Preheat the oven to 350°F (175°C) and grease a muffin tin.
2. In a bowl, whisk together eggs, milk, salt, and pepper.
3. Stir in diced vegetables.
4. Pour the egg mixture evenly into the muffin tin.
5. Bake for 20-25 minutes or until the egg muffins are set and slightly golden.
6. Allow to cool slightly before removing from the muffin tin. Serve warm.

Coconut Chia Seed Pudding:

- Ingredients:
    1. 1/4 cup chia seeds
    2. 1 cup coconut milk
    3. 1 tablespoon honey or maple syrup
    4. 1/2 teaspoon vanilla extract

5. Sliced fruits for topping (such as strawberries, kiwi, or mango)

- ○ Instructions:
    1. In a bowl, whisk together chia seeds, coconut milk, honey or maple syrup, and vanilla extract.
    2. Cover and refrigerate for at least 4 hours or overnight, until the mixture thickens and becomes pudding-like.
    3. Stir well before serving.
    4. Top with sliced fruits and serve chilled.

Cottage Cheese Pancakes:

- ○ Ingredients:
    1. 1 cup cottage cheese
    2. 2 eggs
    3. 1/4 cup flour (all-purpose or oat flour)
    4. 1 teaspoon baking powder

5. 1/2 teaspoon vanilla extract

6. Butter or oil for cooking

- Instructions:

    1. In a blender, combine cottage cheese, eggs, flour, baking powder, and vanilla extract. Blend until smooth.

    2. Heat a non-stick skillet or griddle over medium heat and lightly grease with butter or oil.

    3. Pour batter onto the skillet to form pancakes.

    4. Cook until bubbles form on the surface, then flip and cook until golden brown on the other side.

    5. Serve warm with toppings such as fresh fruit, yogurt, or maple syrup.

Mango Banana Smoothie Bowl:

- Ingredients:
    1. 1 ripe banana
    2. 1 cup frozen mango chunks
    3. 1/2 cup Greek yogurt
    4. 1/4 cup milk (dairy or plant-based)
    5. Toppings: sliced banana, granola, shredded coconut, chia seeds
- Instructions:
    1. In a blender, combine banana, frozen mango chunks, Greek yogurt, and milk. Blend until smooth.
    2. Pour the smoothie into a bowl.
    3. Top with sliced banana, granola, shredded coconut, and chia seeds.
    4. Serve immediately with a spoon.

Vegetable Soup with Quinoa:

- Ingredients:
    1. 1 tablespoon olive oil
    2. 1 onion, diced
    3. 2 carrots, diced
    4. 2 celery stalks, diced
    5. 2 cloves garlic, minced
    6. 1 teaspoon dried thyme
    7. 1/2 cup quinoa, rinsed
    8. 4 cups vegetable broth
    9. Salt and pepper to taste
- Instructions:
    1. Heat olive oil in a large pot over medium heat.
    2. Add diced onion, carrots, and celery. Cook until softened, about 5 minutes.
    3. Stir in minced garlic and dried thyme, cook for another minute.

4. Add quinoa and vegetable broth to the pot. Bring to a boil.
5. Reduce heat and simmer for 15-20 minutes, or until quinoa is cooked.
6. Season with salt and pepper to taste. Serve hot.

Turkey and Avocado Wrap:

- Ingredients:
    1. 2 large whole wheat tortillas
    2. 1/2 lb sliced turkey breast
    3. 1 avocado, sliced
    4. 1 cup baby spinach leaves
    5. 2 tablespoons hummus
- Instructions:
    1. Lay out the tortillas on a flat surface.
    2. Spread hummus evenly on each tortilla.
    3. Layer turkey slices, avocado slices, and

spinach leaves on top of the hummus.

4. Roll up the tortillas tightly, then slice in half diagonally. Serve immediately.

Salmon Salad with Lemon-Dill Dressing:

- Ingredients:
    1. 2 cans (5 oz each) salmon, drained and flaked
    2. 4 cups mixed salad greens
    3. 1 cucumber, sliced
    4. 1/4 red onion, thinly sliced
    5. 1/4 cup chopped fresh dill
    6. 2 tablespoons olive oil
    7. 1 tablespoon lemon juice
    8. Salt and pepper to taste
- Instructions:
    1. In a large bowl, combine salmon, mixed salad greens, sliced cucumber, red onion, and chopped fresh dill.

2. In a small bowl, whisk together olive oil, lemon juice, salt, and pepper to make the dressing.
3. Drizzle the dressing over the salad and toss gently to coat.
4. Divide the salad into individual bowls and serve.

Egg Salad Sandwich:

- Ingredients:
    1. 4 hard-boiled eggs, chopped
    2. 2 tablespoons mayonnaise
    3. 1 tablespoon Dijon mustard
    4. 2 green onions, finely chopped
    5. Salt and pepper to taste
    6. 4 slices whole wheat bread
    7. Lettuce leaves, for serving
- Instructions:

1. In a mixing bowl, combine chopped hard-boiled eggs, mayonnaise, Dijon mustard, chopped green onions, salt, and pepper.
2. Spread the egg salad mixture evenly onto two slices of bread.
3. Top with lettuce leaves and cover with the remaining slices of bread.
4. Slice sandwiches diagonally and serve.

Vegetable Stir-Fry with Tofu:

- Ingredients:
  1. 1 tablespoon sesame oil
  2. 1 block (14 oz) extra-firm tofu, cubed
  3. 2 cups mixed vegetables (bell peppers, broccoli, snap peas, carrots)
  4. 2 cloves garlic, minced
  5. 2 tablespoons soy sauce

6. 1 tablespoon hoisin sauce
7. Cooked rice, for serving

- Instructions:
    1. Heat sesame oil in a large skillet or wok over medium-high heat.
    2. Add cubed tofu to the skillet and cook until golden brown on all sides.
    3. Add mixed vegetables and minced garlic to the skillet. Stir-fry for 3-5 minutes until vegetables are tender-crisp.
    4. Stir in soy sauce and hoisin sauce, tossing to coat evenly.
    5. Serve the vegetable stir-fry over cooked rice.

Mediterranean Chickpea Salad:

- Ingredients:
    1. 1 can (15 oz) chickpeas, drained and rinsed

2. 1 cup cherry tomatoes, halved
3. 1 cucumber, diced
4. 1/4 cup red onion, finely chopped
5. 1/4 cup Kalamata olives, pitted and halved
6. 2 tablespoons chopped fresh parsley
7. 2 tablespoons olive oil
8. 1 tablespoon lemon juice
9. 1 teaspoon dried oregano
10. Salt and pepper to taste

- Instructions:

1. In a large bowl, combine chickpeas, cherry tomatoes, cucumber, red onion, Kalamata olives, and chopped parsley.
2. In a small bowl, whisk together olive oil, lemon juice, dried oregano, salt, and pepper to make the dressing.

3. Drizzle the dressing over the salad and toss gently to coat.
4. Serve chilled.

Chicken and Vegetable Skewers:

- Ingredients:
    1. 1 lb boneless, skinless chicken breast, cut into cubes
    2. 1 bell pepper, cut into chunks
    3. 1 zucchini, sliced
    4. 1 red onion, cut into chunks
    5. 2 tablespoons olive oil
    6. 1 teaspoon garlic powder
    7. 1 teaspoon dried thyme
    8. Salt and pepper to taste
- Instructions:
    1. Preheat grill or grill pan over medium-high heat.
    2. In a bowl, toss chicken cubes, bell pepper chunks,

zucchini slices, and red onion chunks with olive oil, garlic powder, dried thyme, salt, and pepper.

3. Thread the chicken and vegetables onto skewers.
4. Grill skewers for 8-10 minutes, turning occasionally, until chicken is cooked through and vegetables are tender.
5. Serve hot with rice or salad.

Tuna Salad Stuffed Avocado:

- Ingredients:
    1. 2 ripe avocados
    2. 1 can (5 oz) tuna, drained
    3. 1/4 cup diced red bell pepper
    4. 1/4 cup diced cucumber
    5. 2 tablespoons mayonnaise
    6. 1 tablespoon lemon juice
    7. Salt and pepper to taste

- Instructions:
  1. Cut the avocados in half and remove the pits.
  2. In a bowl, combine drained tuna, diced red bell pepper, diced cucumber, mayonnaise, lemon juice, salt, and pepper.
  3. Spoon the tuna salad mixture into the avocado halves.
  4. Serve immediately.

Vegetarian Lentil Soup:

- Ingredients:
  1. 1 tablespoon olive oil
  2. 1 onion, diced
  3. 2 carrots, diced
  4. 2 celery stalks, diced
  5. 2 cloves garlic, minced
  6. 1 cup dried green lentils, rinsed
  7. 4 cups vegetable broth

8. 1 can (14 oz) diced tomatoes
9. 1 teaspoon dried thyme
10. Salt and pepper to taste

- Instructions:
    1. Heat olive oil in a large pot over medium heat.
    2. Add diced onion, carrots, celery, and minced garlic. Cook until softened, about 5 minutes.
    3. Stir in dried green lentils, vegetable broth, diced tomatoes, and dried thyme.
    4. Bring to a boil, then reduce heat and simmer for 25-30 minutes, or until lentils are tender.
    5. Season with salt and pepper to taste. Serve hot.

Caprese Salad with Balsamic Glaze:

- Ingredients:

1. 2 large tomatoes, sliced
        2. 1 ball fresh mozzarella cheese, sliced
        3. Fresh basil leaves
        4. Balsamic glaze
        5. Salt and pepper to taste
- Instructions:
        1. Arrange tomato slices and mozzarella slices on a serving platter, alternating them.
        2. Tuck fresh basil leaves between the tomato and mozzarella slices.
        3. Drizzle balsamic glaze over the salad.
        4. Season with salt and pepper to taste. Serve immediately.

Baked Salmon with Roasted Vegetables:

- Ingredients:
    1. 2 salmon fillets
    2. 2 tablespoons olive oil
    3. 1 teaspoon lemon juice
    4. Salt and pepper to taste
    5. 2 cups mixed vegetables (such as broccoli, bell peppers, carrots)
    6. 1 tablespoon balsamic vinegar
    7. 1 teaspoon dried herbs (such as thyme or rosemary)
- Instructions:
    1. Preheat the oven to 400°F (200°C).
    2. Place salmon fillets on a baking sheet lined with parchment paper.
    3. Drizzle olive oil and lemon juice over the salmon, then

season with salt and pepper.

4. In a separate bowl, toss mixed vegetables with olive oil, balsamic vinegar, dried herbs, salt, and pepper.
5. Spread the vegetables around the salmon on the baking sheet.
6. Bake in the preheated oven for 15-20 minutes, or until salmon is cooked through and vegetables are tender.

Turkey and Vegetable Stir-Fry:

- Ingredients:
    1. 1 lb ground turkey
    2. 2 tablespoons soy sauce
    3. 1 tablespoon sesame oil
    4. 2 cloves garlic, minced
    5. 1 teaspoon grated ginger

6. 2 cups mixed vegetables (such as bell peppers, snap peas, carrots)
7. Cooked rice, for serving

- Instructions:
  1. Heat sesame oil in a large skillet or wok over medium heat.
  2. Add ground turkey to the skillet and cook until browned.
  3. Stir in minced garlic and grated ginger, cook for another minute.
  4. Add mixed vegetables to the skillet and stir-fry until tender-crisp.
  5. Drizzle soy sauce over the turkey and vegetables, tossing to coat evenly.
  6. Serve the turkey and vegetable stir-fry over cooked rice.

Pasta Primavera:

- Ingredients:
    1. 8 oz pasta (such as penne or spaghetti)
    2. 2 tablespoons olive oil
    3. 2 cloves garlic, minced
    4. 2 cups mixed vegetables (such as cherry tomatoes, zucchini, bell peppers)
    5. 1/4 cup grated Parmesan cheese
    6. Salt and pepper to taste
    7. Fresh basil leaves, for garnish
- Instructions:
    1. Cook pasta according to package instructions until al dente. Drain and set aside.
    2. Heat olive oil in a large skillet over medium heat.
    3. Add minced garlic to the skillet and cook until fragrant.

4. Add mixed vegetables to the skillet and sauté until tender.
5. Toss cooked pasta with the vegetables in the skillet.
6. Sprinkle grated Parmesan cheese over the pasta and vegetables, season with salt and pepper.
7. Garnish with fresh basil leaves before serving.

Slow Cooker Chicken and Vegetable Soup:

- Ingredients:
    1. 1 lb boneless, skinless chicken thighs
    2. 4 cups chicken broth
    3. 2 carrots, diced
    4. 2 celery stalks, diced
    5. 1 onion, diced
    6. 2 cloves garlic, minced
    7. 1 teaspoon dried thyme
    8. Salt and pepper to taste

- o Instructions:
    1. Place chicken thighs in the slow cooker.
    2. Add diced carrots, celery, onion, minced garlic, dried thyme, salt, and pepper.
    3. Pour chicken broth over the ingredients in the slow cooker.
    4. Cover and cook on low for 6-8 hours or on high for 3-4 hours, until chicken is cooked through and vegetables are tender.
    5. Shred the chicken with forks before serving.

Vegetarian Bean Chili:

- o Ingredients:
    1. 2 tablespoons olive oil
    2. 1 onion, diced
    3. 2 bell peppers, diced
    4. 2 cloves garlic, minced
    5. 2 teaspoons chili powder

6. 1 teaspoon ground cumin
7. 1 can (15 oz) black beans, drained and rinsed
8. 1 can (15 oz) kidney beans, drained and rinsed
9. 1 can (14 oz) diced tomatoes
10. 2 cups vegetable broth
11. Salt and pepper to taste
- Instructions:
    1. Heat olive oil in a large pot over medium heat.
    2. Add diced onion and bell peppers to the pot, sauté until softened.
    3. Stir in minced garlic, chili powder, and ground cumin, cook for another minute.
    4. Add black beans, kidney beans, diced tomatoes, and vegetable broth to the pot.
    5. Bring to a boil, then reduce heat and simmer

for 20-30 minutes, stirring occasionally.
6. Season with salt and pepper to taste. Serve hot.

Baked Chicken and Vegetables:

- Ingredients:
    1. 2 boneless, skinless chicken breasts
    2. 2 tablespoons olive oil
    3. 1 teaspoon garlic powder
    4. 1 teaspoon dried Italian seasoning
    5. Salt and pepper to taste
    6. 2 cups mixed vegetables (such as potatoes, carrots, green beans)
- Instructions:
    1. Preheat the oven to 400°F (200°C).
    2. Place chicken breasts in a baking dish and drizzle with olive oil.

3. Season chicken with garlic powder, dried Italian seasoning, salt, and pepper.
4. Arrange mixed vegetables around the chicken in the baking dish.
5. Bake for 20-25 minutes, or until chicken is cooked through and vegetables are tender.

Shrimp Stir-Fry with Brown Rice:

- Ingredients:
    1. 1 lb large shrimp, peeled and deveined
    2. 2 tablespoons soy sauce
    3. 1 tablespoon sesame oil
    4. 2 cloves garlic, minced
    5. 1 teaspoon grated ginger
    6. 2 cups mixed vegetables (such as broccoli, bell peppers, snap peas)

7. Cooked brown rice, for serving

- o Instructions:
    1. In a bowl, marinate shrimp in soy sauce and sesame oil for 15 minutes.
    2. Heat olive oil in a large skillet or wok over medium heat.
    3. Add minced garlic and grated ginger to the skillet and cook until fragrant.
    4. Add marinated shrimp to the skillet and stir-fry until pink and cooked through.
    5. Stir in mixed vegetables and continue to cook until tender-crisp.
    6. Serve shrimp and vegetables over cooked brown rice.

Vegetable and Bean Quesadillas:

- o Ingredients:

1. 4 large whole wheat tortillas
2. 1 can (15 oz) black beans, drained and rinsed
3. 1 cup shredded cheese (cheddar or Mexican blend)
4. 1 cup mixed vegetables (such as bell peppers, onions, corn)
5. 1 teaspoon chili powder
6. 1/2 teaspoon ground cumin
7. Salt and pepper to taste

- Instructions:
  1. In a bowl, mash black beans with chili powder, ground cumin, salt, and pepper.
  2. Spread mashed black beans evenly onto two tortillas.

3. Top each tortilla with shredded cheese and mixed vegetables.
4. Place another tortilla on top to cover the filling, forming a quesadilla.
5. Heat a skillet over medium heat and cook quesadillas for 2-3 minutes on each side, until golden brown and cheese is melted.
6. Cut quesadillas into wedges and serve with salsa or guacamole.

Lemon Herb Baked Cod:

- Ingredients:
    1. 4 cod fillets
    2. 2 tablespoons olive oil
    3. 2 tablespoons lemon juice
    4. 2 cloves garlic, minced
    5. 1 teaspoon dried thyme
    6. 1 teaspoon dried parsley
    7. Salt and pepper to taste

- Instructions:
    1. Preheat the oven to 400°F (200°C).
    2. Place cod fillets in a baking dish and drizzle with olive oil and lemon juice.
    3. Sprinkle minced garlic, dried thyme, dried parsley, salt, and pepper over the cod fillets.
    4. Bake for 15-20 minutes, or until fish is opaque and flakes easily with a fork.

Vegetarian Stuffed Bell Peppers:

- Ingredients:
    1. 4 bell peppers, halved and seeds removed
    2. 1 cup cooked quinoa
    3. 1 can (15 oz) black beans, drained and rinsed
    4. 1 cup corn kernels
    5. 1 cup diced tomatoes
    6. 1 teaspoon chili powder

7. 1/2 teaspoon ground cumin
8. Salt and pepper to taste
9. 1/2 cup shredded cheese (optional)

○ Instructions:

1. Preheat the oven to 375°F (190°C).
2. In a bowl, combine cooked quinoa, black beans, corn kernels, diced tomatoes, chili powder, ground cumin, salt, and pepper.
3. Stuff each bell pepper half with the quinoa and bean mixture.
4. Place stuffed bell peppers in a baking dish and cover with foil.
5. Bake for 25-30 minutes, or until peppers are tender.
6. If desired, sprinkle shredded cheese over the stuffed peppers during the

last 5 minutes of baking until melted.
7. Serve hot.

Chapter 9:SOUPS AND STEWS RECIPES

Chicken and Vegetable Soup:

- Ingredients:
    1. 1 tablespoon olive oil
    2. 2 boneless, skinless chicken breasts, diced
    3. 1 onion, chopped
    4. 2 carrots, diced
    5. 2 celery stalks, diced
    6. 2 cloves garlic, minced
    7. 6 cups chicken broth
    8. 1 teaspoon dried thyme
    9. Salt and pepper to taste
- Instructions:
    1. Heat olive oil in a large pot over medium heat.

2. Add diced chicken breast to the pot and cook until browned.
3. Add chopped onion, diced carrots, diced celery, and minced garlic to the pot. Cook until vegetables are softened.
4. Pour chicken broth into the pot and bring to a boil.
5. Reduce heat to low, add dried thyme, salt, and pepper. Simmer for 20-25 minutes.
6. Serve hot.

Vegetable Lentil Soup:

- Ingredients:
    1. 1 tablespoon olive oil
    2. 1 onion, chopped
    3. 2 carrots, diced
    4. 2 celery stalks, diced
    5. 2 cloves garlic, minced
    6. 1 cup dried lentils, rinsed

7. 6 cups vegetable broth
8. 1 can (14 oz) diced tomatoes
9. 1 teaspoon dried thyme
10. Salt and pepper to taste

- Instructions:
    1. Heat olive oil in a large pot over medium heat.
    2. Add chopped onion, diced carrots, diced celery, and minced garlic to the pot. Cook until vegetables are softened.
    3. Stir in dried lentils, vegetable broth, diced tomatoes, and dried thyme. Bring to a boil.
    4. Reduce heat to low, cover, and simmer for 25-30 minutes, or until lentils are tender.
    5. Season with salt and pepper to taste. Serve hot.

Beef and Barley Stew:

- Ingredients:
    1. 1 tablespoon olive oil
    2. 1 lb beef stew meat, cubed
    3. 1 onion, chopped
    4. 2 carrots, diced
    5. 2 celery stalks, diced
    6. 2 cloves garlic, minced
    7. 6 cups beef broth
    8. 1 cup pearl barley
    9. 1 teaspoon dried thyme
    10. Salt and pepper to taste
- Instructions:
    1. Heat olive oil in a large pot over medium heat.
    2. Add cubed beef stew meat to the pot and cook until browned.
    3. Add chopped onion, diced carrots, diced celery, and minced garlic to the pot. Cook until vegetables are softened.

4. Pour beef broth into the pot and bring to a boil.
5. Stir in pearl barley and dried thyme. Reduce heat to low, cover, and simmer for 45-50 minutes, or until barley is tender.
6. Season with salt and pepper to taste. Serve hot.

Tomato Basil Soup:

- Ingredients:
    1. 1 tablespoon olive oil
    2. 1 onion, chopped
    3. 2 cloves garlic, minced
    4. 2 cans (14 oz each) diced tomatoes
    5. 4 cups vegetable broth
    6. 1/4 cup chopped fresh basil leaves
    7. Salt and pepper to taste
- Instructions:
    1. Heat olive oil in a large pot over medium heat.

2. Add chopped onion and minced garlic to the pot. Cook until softened.

3. Stir in diced tomatoes (with their juices) and vegetable broth. Bring to a boil.

4. Reduce heat to low and simmer for 15-20 minutes.

5. Use an immersion blender to blend the soup until smooth.

6. Stir in chopped fresh basil leaves. Season with salt and pepper to taste. Serve hot.

Potato Leek Soup:

o Ingredients:

1. 2 tablespoons butter

2. 2 leeks, white and light green parts only, sliced

3. 3 potatoes, peeled and diced

4. 4 cups vegetable broth
5. 1 cup milk (dairy or plant-based)
6. Salt and pepper to taste
- Instructions:
    1. In a large pot, melt butter over medium heat.
    2. Add sliced leeks to the pot and cook until softened.
    3. Stir in diced potatoes and vegetable broth. Bring to a boil.
    4. Reduce heat to low, cover, and simmer for 20-25 minutes, or until potatoes are tender.
    5. Use an immersion blender to blend the soup until smooth.
    6. Stir in milk and heat through. Season with salt and pepper to taste. Serve hot.

Butternut Squash Soup:

- Ingredients:
    1. 1 butternut squash, peeled, seeded, and diced
    2. 1 onion, chopped
    3. 2 carrots, diced
    4. 2 cloves garlic, minced
    5. 4 cups vegetable broth
    6. 1 teaspoon ground ginger
    7. 1/2 teaspoon ground cinnamon
    8. Salt and pepper to taste
- Instructions:
    1. In a large pot, combine diced butternut squash, chopped onion, diced carrots, minced garlic, and vegetable broth.
    2. Bring to a boil, then reduce heat to low and simmer for 20-25 minutes, or until vegetables are tender.

3. Use an immersion blender to blend the soup until smooth.
4. Stir in ground ginger and ground cinnamon. Season with salt and pepper to taste. Serve hot.

Creamy Mushroom Soup:

- o Ingredients:
  1. 2 tablespoons butter
  2. 1 onion, chopped
  3. 2 cloves garlic, minced
  4. 16 oz mushrooms, sliced
  5. 4 cups vegetable broth
  6. 1 cup heavy cream
  7. Salt and pepper to taste
- o Instructions:
  1. In a large pot, melt butter over medium heat.
  2. Add chopped onion and minced garlic to the pot. Cook until softened.

3. Add sliced mushrooms to the pot and cook until they release their juices.
4. Pour vegetable broth into the pot and bring to a boil.
5. Reduce heat to low, cover, and simmer for 15-20 minutes.
6. Use an immersion blender to blend the soup until smooth.
7. Stir in heavy cream and heat through. Season with salt and pepper to taste. Serve hot.

Chicken and Rice Soup:

- Ingredients:
  1. 1 tablespoon olive oil
  2. 2 boneless, skinless chicken breasts, diced
  3. 1 onion, chopped
  4. 2 carrots, diced
  5. 2 celery stalks, diced

6. 2 cloves garlic, minced
7. 6 cups chicken broth
8. 1 cup cooked rice
9. 1 teaspoon dried thyme
10. Salt and pepper to taste

- Instructions:
    1. Heat olive oil in a large pot over medium heat.
    2. Add diced chicken breast to the pot and cook until browned.
    3. Add chopped onion, diced carrots, diced celery, and minced garlic to the pot. Cook until vegetables are softened.
    4. Pour chicken broth into the pot and bring to a boil.
    5. Stir in cooked rice and dried thyme. Reduce heat to low, cover, and simmer for 20-25 minutes.
    6. Season with salt and pepper to taste. Serve hot.

Split Pea Soup:

- Ingredients:
    1. 1 tablespoon olive oil
    2. 1 onion, chopped
    3. 2 carrots, diced
    4. 2 celery stalks, diced
    5. 2 cloves garlic, minced
    6. 1 lb dried split peas, rinsed
    7. 8 cups vegetable broth
    8. 1 bay leaf
    9. Salt and pepper to taste
- Instructions:
    1. Heat olive oil in a large pot over medium heat.
    2. Add chopped onion, diced carrots, diced celery, and minced garlic to the pot. Cook until softened.
    3. Stir in dried split peas, vegetable broth, and bay leaf. Bring to a boil.
    4. Reduce heat to low, cover, and simmer for 1 to 1 1/2

hours, or until peas are tender.

5. Remove bay leaf and use an immersion blender to blend the soup until smooth (or leave it chunky if preferred).

6. Season with salt and pepper to taste. Serve hot.

Vegetable Minestrone Soup:

- Ingredients:
    1. 1 tablespoon olive oil
    2. 1 onion, chopped
    3. 2 carrots, diced
    4. 2 celery stalks, diced
    5. 2 cloves garlic, minced
    6. 1 can (14 oz) diced tomatoes
    7. 6 cups vegetable broth
    8. 1 cup small pasta (such as ditalini or elbow macaroni)

9. 1 can (15 oz) kidney beans, drained and rinsed
10.   1 teaspoon dried basil
11. Salt and pepper to taste
- Instructions:
    1. Heat olive oil in a large pot over medium heat.
    2. Add chopped onion, diced carrots, diced celery, and minced garlic to the pot. Cook until softened.
    3. Stir in diced tomatoes, vegetable broth, and small pasta. Bring to a boil.
    4. Reduce heat to low, cover, and simmer for 10 minutes.
    5. Stir in kidney beans and dried basil. Simmer for another 5-10 minutes, or until pasta is cooked.
    6. Season with salt and pepper to taste. Serve hot.

Chapter 10:SALADS AND SIDES RECIPES

Quinoa Salad with Chickpeas and Vegetables:

- Ingredients:
    1. 1 cup quinoa, rinsed
    2. 1 can (15 oz) chickpeas, drained and rinsed
    3. 1 cucumber, diced
    4. 1 bell pepper, diced
    5. 1/4 cup chopped fresh parsley
    6. 2 tablespoons olive oil
    7. 1 tablespoon lemon juice
    8. Salt and pepper to taste
- Instructions:
    1. Cook quinoa according to package instructions. Let it cool.
    2. In a large bowl, combine cooked quinoa, chickpeas, diced cucumber, diced bell

pepper, and chopped fresh parsley.

3. In a small bowl, whisk together olive oil, lemon juice, salt, and pepper.
4. Pour the dressing over the quinoa salad and toss gently to combine.
5. Serve chilled.

Roasted Sweet Potato Wedges:

- Ingredients:
    1. 2 sweet potatoes, scrubbed and cut into wedges
    2. 2 tablespoons olive oil
    3. 1 teaspoon paprika
    4. 1/2 teaspoon garlic powder
    5. Salt and pepper to taste
- Instructions:
    1. Preheat the oven to 400°F (200°C).
    2. In a large bowl, toss sweet potato wedges with olive oil, paprika, garlic powder,

salt, and pepper until evenly coated.

3. Arrange the sweet potato wedges in a single layer on a baking sheet lined with parchment paper.
4. Bake for 25-30 minutes, flipping halfway through, until tender and golden brown.
5. Serve hot as a side dish.

Spinach and Strawberry Salad with Balsamic Vinaigrette:

- Ingredients:
    1. 4 cups baby spinach leaves
    2. 1 cup sliced strawberries
    3. 1/4 cup chopped pecans
    4. 2 tablespoons crumbled feta cheese (optional)
    5. 2 tablespoons balsamic vinegar
    6. 1 tablespoon olive oil
    7. 1 teaspoon honey

8. Salt and pepper to taste

- Instructions:
    1. In a large bowl, combine baby spinach leaves, sliced strawberries, chopped pecans, and crumbled feta cheese.
    2. In a small bowl, whisk together balsamic vinegar, olive oil, honey, salt, and pepper to make the dressing.
    3. Drizzle the dressing over the salad and toss gently to coat.
    4. Serve immediately.

Cucumber and Tomato Salad:

- Ingredients:
    1. 2 cucumbers, thinly sliced
    2. 2 tomatoes, diced
    3. 1/4 cup thinly sliced red onion

4. 2 tablespoons chopped fresh dill
5. 2 tablespoons olive oil
6. 1 tablespoon red wine vinegar
7. Salt and pepper to taste
- Instructions:
1. In a large bowl, combine thinly sliced cucumbers, diced tomatoes, thinly sliced red onion, and chopped fresh dill.
2. In a small bowl, whisk together olive oil, red wine vinegar, salt, and pepper to make the dressing.
3. Drizzle the dressing over the salad and toss gently to coat.
4. Serve chilled.

Garlic Herb Roasted Potatoes:

- Ingredients:
1. 1 lb baby potatoes, halved

2. 2 tablespoons olive oil
3. 2 cloves garlic, minced
4. 1 teaspoon dried thyme
5. 1 teaspoon dried rosemary
6. Salt and pepper to taste

- Instructions:
    1. Preheat the oven to 400°F (200°C).
    2. In a large bowl, toss halved baby potatoes with olive oil, minced garlic, dried thyme, dried rosemary, salt, and pepper until evenly coated.
    3. Arrange the potatoes in a single layer on a baking sheet lined with parchment paper.
    4. Bake for 25-30 minutes, flipping halfway through, until golden brown and crispy.
    5. Serve hot as a side dish.

Broccoli Salad with Bacon and Cranberries:

- Ingredients:
    1. 4 cups broccoli florets
    2. 4 slices bacon, cooked and crumbled
    3. 1/4 cup dried cranberries
    4. 1/4 cup chopped red onion
    5. 1/4 cup sunflower seeds
    6. 1/2 cup mayonnaise
    7. 2 tablespoons apple cider vinegar
    8. 1 tablespoon honey
    9. Salt and pepper to taste
- Instructions:
    1. In a large bowl, combine broccoli florets, crumbled bacon, dried cranberries, chopped red onion, and sunflower seeds.
    2. In a small bowl, whisk together mayonnaise, apple cider vinegar, honey,

salt, and pepper to make the dressing.
3. Pour the dressing over the salad and toss gently to coat.
4. Serve chilled.

Mashed Cauliflower with Garlic and Parmesan:

- Ingredients:
    1. 1 head cauliflower, chopped into florets
    2. 2 cloves garlic, minced
    3. 2 tablespoons butter
    4. 1/4 cup grated Parmesan cheese
    5. Salt and pepper to taste
- Instructions:
    1. Steam or boil cauliflower florets until tender, about 10-15 minutes.
    2. Drain the cauliflower and transfer to a food processor.

3. Add minced garlic, butter, grated Parmesan cheese, salt, and pepper to the food processor.
4. Blend until smooth and creamy.
5. Adjust seasoning if needed and serve hot.

Caprese Pasta Salad:

- Ingredients:
    1. 8 oz pasta (such as penne or fusilli)
    2. 1 cup cherry tomatoes, halved
    3. 1 ball fresh mozzarella cheese, diced
    4. 1/4 cup chopped fresh basil leaves
    5. 2 tablespoons olive oil
    6. 1 tablespoon balsamic vinegar
    7. Salt and pepper to taste
- Instructions:

1. Cook pasta according to package instructions until al dente. Drain and let it cool.
2. In a large bowl, combine cooked pasta, halved cherry tomatoes, diced fresh mozzarella cheese, and chopped fresh basil leaves.
3. Drizzle olive oil and balsamic vinegar over the salad.
4. Season with salt and pepper to taste. Toss gently to combine.
5. Serve chilled.

Green Bean Almondine:

- Ingredients:
  1. 1 lb green beans, trimmed
  2. 2 tablespoons butter
  3. 1/4 cup sliced almonds
  4. 1 tablespoon lemon juice

5. Salt and pepper to taste

- o Instructions:
    1. Steam or boil green beans until tender-crisp, about 5-7 minutes. Drain and set aside.
    2. In a large skillet, melt butter over medium heat.
    3. Add sliced almonds to the skillet and cook until lightly toasted.
    4. Add cooked green beans to the skillet and toss to coat with butter and almonds.
    5. Drizzle lemon juice over the green beans. Season with salt and pepper to taste. Serve hot.

Greek Cucumber Salad:

- o Ingredients:
    1. 2 cucumbers, thinly sliced
    2. 1/4 cup sliced red onion

3. 1/4 cup Kalamata olives, pitted and halved
4. 1/4 cup crumbled feta cheese
5. 2 tablespoons chopped fresh dill
6. 2 tablespoons olive oil
7. 1 tablespoon red wine vinegar
8. Salt and pepper to taste
- Instructions:
    1. In a large bowl, combine thinly sliced cucumbers, sliced red onion, halved Kalamata olives, crumbled feta cheese, and chopped fresh dill.
    2. In a small bowl, whisk together olive oil, red wine vinegar, salt, and pepper to make the dressing.
    3. Drizzle the dressing over the salad and toss gently to coat.

4. Serve chilled.

Chapter 11: VEGETARIAN MAINS RECIPES

1. **Quinoa-Stuffed Bell Peppers:**
   - Ingredients:
     1. 4 large bell peppers
     2. 1 cup quinoa
     3. 2 cups vegetable broth
     4. 1 can black beans, drained and rinsed
     5. 1 cup corn kernels
     6. 1 cup diced tomatoes
     7. 1 teaspoon cumin
     8. 1 teaspoon chili powder
     9. Salt and pepper to taste
   - Instructions:
     1. Preheat oven to 375°F (190°C).
     2. Cook quinoa according to package instructions, using vegetable broth for extra flavor.

3. In a large bowl, mix cooked quinoa, black beans, corn, diced tomatoes, cumin, chili powder, salt, and pepper.
4. Cut the tops off the bell peppers and remove seeds and membranes.
5. Stuff each pepper with the quinoa mixture.
6. Place stuffed peppers in a baking dish and cover with foil.
7. Bake for 25-30 minutes until peppers are tender.
8. Serve hot.

Vegetable Stir-Fry with Tofu:

- Ingredients:
    1. 1 block tofu, pressed and cubed
    2. 2 cups mixed vegetables (such as bell peppers,

broccoli, carrots, snap peas)

3. 2 cloves garlic, minced
4. 1 tablespoon ginger, minced
5. 2 tablespoons soy sauce
6. 1 tablespoon sesame oil
7. 1 tablespoon olive oil
8. Cooked rice or noodles, for serving

- Instructions:
  1. Heat olive oil in a large skillet over medium heat.
  2. Add tofu cubes and cook until golden brown on all sides. Remove from skillet and set aside.
  3. In the same skillet, add sesame oil and sauté garlic and ginger until fragrant.
  4. Add mixed vegetables and stir-fry until crisp-tender.

5. Return tofu to the skillet and add soy sauce. Stir well to combine.
6. Serve hot over cooked rice or noodles.

Spinach and Mushroom Quiche:

- Ingredients:
  1. 1 pre-made pie crust
  2. 1 cup chopped spinach
  3. 1 cup sliced mushrooms
  4. 1 onion, diced
  5. 4 eggs
  6. 1 cup milk or non-dairy milk
  7. 1 cup shredded cheese (optional)
  8. Salt and pepper to taste
- Instructions:
  1. Preheat oven to 375°F (190°C).
  2. In a skillet, sauté onions until translucent. Add mushrooms and spinach,

and cook until vegetables are tender. Remove from heat.

3. In a bowl, whisk together eggs, milk, salt, and pepper.
4. Place the pre-made pie crust in a pie dish.
5. Spread the cooked vegetables evenly over the pie crust.
6. Pour the egg mixture over the vegetables.
7. Sprinkle shredded cheese on top if using.
8. Bake for 35-40 minutes until the quiche is set and golden brown.
9. Let it cool slightly before slicing and serving.

Vegetable Lentil Soup:

- Ingredients:
  1. 1 cup dry lentils, rinsed

2. 4 cups vegetable broth
3. 1 onion, diced
4. 2 carrots, diced
5. 2 celery stalks, diced
6. 2 cloves garlic, minced
7. 1 can diced tomatoes
8. 1 teaspoon dried thyme
9. Salt and pepper to taste

- Instructions:
    1. In a large pot, combine lentils, vegetable broth, onion, carrots, celery, garlic, diced tomatoes, thyme, salt, and pepper.
    2. Bring to a boil, then reduce heat and let simmer for 30-40 minutes until lentils and vegetables are tender.
    3. Adjust seasoning if needed.
    4. Serve hot with crusty bread on the side.

Eggplant Parmesan:

- Ingredients:
    1. 2 medium eggplants, sliced into rounds
    2. 2 cups marinara sauce
    3. 1 cup breadcrumbs
    4. 1 cup grated Parmesan cheese
    5. 2 eggs, beaten
    6. 2 cups shredded mozzarella cheese
    7. Salt and pepper to taste
    8. Olive oil for frying
- Instructions:
    1. Preheat oven to 375°F (190°C).
    2. Season eggplant slices with salt and let sit for 10 minutes to draw out moisture. Pat dry with paper towels.
    3. Dip eggplant slices in beaten eggs, then coat with

breadcrumbs mixed with grated Parmesan cheese.

4. Heat olive oil in a skillet over medium heat. Fry eggplant slices until golden brown on both sides. Remove from skillet and drain excess oil on paper towels.
5. Spread a thin layer of marinara sauce in the bottom of a baking dish.
6. Arrange fried eggplant slices in the baking dish, overlapping slightly.
7. Top eggplant slices with remaining marinara sauce and shredded mozzarella cheese.
8. Bake for 25-30 minutes until cheese is bubbly and golden brown.
9. Let it cool slightly before serving.

Vegetable Paella:

- Ingredients:
    1. 1 cup Arborio rice
    2. 2 cups vegetable broth
    3. 1 onion, diced
    4. 2 cloves garlic, minced
    5. 1 red bell pepper, sliced
    6. 1 yellow bell pepper, sliced
    7. 1 cup frozen peas
    8. 1 tomato, diced
    9. 1 teaspoon smoked paprika
    10. Pinch of saffron threads (optional)
    11. Salt and pepper to taste
    12. Olive oil for cooking
- Instructions:
    1. Heat olive oil in a large skillet or paella pan over medium heat.
    2. Sauté onions and garlic until translucent.
    3. Add bell peppers and cook until slightly softened.

4. Stir in Arborio rice and cook for a few minutes until lightly toasted.
5. Pour in vegetable broth and add saffron threads if using. Season with smoked paprika, salt, and pepper.
6. Bring to a simmer, then reduce heat to low and cover. Let cook for 15-20 minutes until rice is tender and liquid is absorbed.
7. Stir in frozen peas and diced tomatoes. Cook for an additional 5 minutes until peas are heated through.
8. Serve hot, garnished with fresh parsley if desired.

Vegetarian Chili:

- Ingredients:
  1. 2 cans kidney beans, drained and rinsed

2. 1 can black beans, drained and rinsed
3. 1 onion, diced
4. 2 cloves garlic, minced
5. 1 bell pepper, diced
6. 1 zucchini, diced
7. 1 can diced tomatoes
8. 1 cup vegetable broth
9. 2 tablespoons chili powder
10. 1 teaspoon cumin
11. Salt and pepper to taste
12. Olive oil for cooking

- Instructions:
  1. Heat olive oil in a large pot over medium heat.
  2. Sauté onions and garlic until softened.
  3. Add bell pepper and zucchini, and cook until vegetables are tender.
  4. Stir in chili powder and cumin, and cook for another minute until fragrant.

5. Add diced tomatoes, vegetable broth, kidney beans, and black beans. Season with salt and pepper.
6. Bring to a simmer, then reduce heat to low and let chili cook for 20-25 minutes, stirring occasionally.
7. Adjust seasoning if needed.
8. Serve hot, optionally garnished with shredded cheese, sour cream, or chopped cilantro.

Mushroom Risotto:

- Ingredients:
    1. 1 cup Arborio rice
    2. 4 cups vegetable broth
    3. 2 tablespoons olive oil
    4. 1 onion, diced
    5. 2 cloves garlic, minced

6. 2 cups sliced mushrooms (such as cremini or shiitake)
7. 1/2 cup dry white wine (optional)
8. 1/2 cup grated Parmesan cheese
9. Salt and pepper to taste

- Instructions:
    1. In a saucepan, heat vegetable broth and keep it warm over low heat.
    2. In a separate large skillet, heat olive oil over medium heat. Add onions and garlic, and sauté until translucent.
    3. Add sliced mushrooms and cook until they release their moisture and become tender.
    4. Stir in Arborio rice and cook for a few minutes until lightly toasted.

5. If using wine, pour it into the skillet and cook until it's absorbed by the rice.
6. Gradually add warm vegetable broth to the skillet, one ladleful at a time, stirring constantly and allowing the liquid to absorb before adding more.
7. Continue cooking and stirring until the rice is creamy and tender, about 20-25 minutes.
8. Stir in grated Parmesan cheese and season with salt and pepper.
9. Serve hot, optionally garnished with chopped parsley.

Vegetable Curry:

- Ingredients:

1. 2 cups mixed vegetables (such as cauliflower, carrots, potatoes, peas)
2. 1 onion, diced
3. 2 cloves garlic, minced
4. 1 tablespoon ginger, minced
5. 1 can coconut milk
6. 2 tablespoons curry powder
7. 1 tablespoon tomato paste
8. 1 tablespoon olive oil
9. Salt and pepper to taste

- Instructions:
    1. Heat olive oil in a large skillet over medium heat.
    2. Sauté onions, garlic, and ginger until softened and fragrant.
    3. Add mixed vegetables to the skillet and cook until they begin to soften.

4. Stir in curry powder and tomato paste, and cook for another minute.
5. Pour in coconut milk and bring to a simmer. Let curry simmer for 15-20 minutes until vegetables are tender and the sauce has thickened.
6. Season with salt and pepper to taste.
7. Serve hot over cooked rice or quinoa.

Caprese Pasta Salad:

- Ingredients:
    1. 8 oz pasta (such as fusilli or penne)
    2. 1 cup cherry tomatoes, halved
    3. 1 ball fresh mozzarella cheese, diced
    4. 1/4 cup fresh basil leaves, chopped

5. 2 tablespoons balsamic vinegar
6. 2 tablespoons olive oil
7. Salt and pepper to taste
- Instructions:
  1. Cook pasta according to package instructions. Drain and rinse under cold water to cool.
  2. In a large bowl, combine cooked pasta, cherry tomatoes, diced mozzarella, and chopped basil.
  3. Drizzle balsamic vinegar and olive oil over the pasta salad. Season with salt and pepper.
  4. Toss everything together until well combined.
  5. Serve chilled or at room temperature.

Baked Lemon Herb Chicken:

- Ingredients:
    1. 4 boneless, skinless chicken breasts
    2. 2 tablespoons olive oil
    3. 2 cloves garlic, minced
    4. Zest and juice of 1 lemon
    5. 1 teaspoon dried thyme
    6. 1 teaspoon dried rosemary
    7. Salt and pepper to taste
- Instructions:
    1. Preheat oven to 375°F (190°C).
    2. In a small bowl, whisk together olive oil, minced garlic, lemon zest, lemon juice, dried thyme, dried rosemary, salt, and pepper.
    3. Place chicken breasts in a baking dish and pour the

lemon herb mixture over them, ensuring they are evenly coated.

4. Bake in the preheated oven for 25-30 minutes, or until the chicken is cooked through and no longer pink in the center.
5. Serve hot, garnished with additional lemon slices if desired.

Salmon with Dill Sauce:

- Ingredients:
    1. 4 salmon fillets
    2. Salt and pepper to taste
    3. 2 tablespoons olive oil
    4. 1/4 cup Greek yogurt
    5. 2 tablespoons chopped fresh dill
    6. 1 tablespoon Dijon mustard
    7. 1 tablespoon lemon juice
- Instructions:

1. Season salmon fillets with salt and pepper.
2. Heat olive oil in a skillet over medium-high heat.
3. Place salmon fillets in the skillet and cook for 4-5 minutes per side, or until salmon is cooked through and flakes easily with a fork.
4. In a small bowl, whisk together Greek yogurt, chopped dill, Dijon mustard, and lemon juice to make the dill sauce.
5. Serve cooked salmon hot, topped with dill sauce.

Turkey Vegetable Stir-Fry:

- Ingredients:
  1. 1 lb turkey breast, thinly sliced
  2. 2 tablespoons soy sauce
  3. 1 tablespoon olive oil

4. 2 cloves garlic, minced
5. 1 onion, sliced
6. 2 cups mixed vegetables (such as bell peppers, broccoli, carrots)
7. Cooked rice or noodles, for serving

- Instructions:
    1. In a bowl, marinate thinly sliced turkey breast in soy sauce for 15-20 minutes.
    2. Heat olive oil in a large skillet or wok over medium-high heat.
    3. Add minced garlic and sliced onion to the skillet, and cook until softened and fragrant.
    4. Add marinated turkey slices to the skillet and stir-fry until cooked through.
    5. Add mixed vegetables to the skillet and continue

stir-frying until vegetables are tender-crisp.

6. Serve hot over cooked rice or noodles.

Lemon Garlic Shrimp Pasta:

- Ingredients:
    1. 8 oz pasta (such as linguine or spaghetti)
    2. 1 lb large shrimp, peeled and deveined
    3. Salt and pepper to taste
    4. 2 tablespoons olive oil
    5. 4 cloves garlic, minced
    6. Zest and juice of 1 lemon
    7. 1/4 cup chopped fresh parsley
- Instructions:
    1. Cook pasta according to package instructions. Drain and set aside.
    2. Season shrimp with salt and pepper.

3. Heat olive oil in a large skillet over medium heat.
4. Add minced garlic to the skillet and cook until fragrant, about 1 minute.
5. Add seasoned shrimp to the skillet and cook until pink and opaque, about 2-3 minutes per side.
6. Stir in lemon zest and lemon juice, then add cooked pasta to the skillet. Toss everything together until well combined.
7. Remove from heat and sprinkle chopped parsley over the pasta.
8. Serve hot.

Coconut Curry Chicken:

- Ingredients:
  1. 4 boneless, skinless chicken breasts, cut into bite-sized pieces

2. 1 tablespoon olive oil
3. 1 onion, diced
4. 2 cloves garlic, minced
5. 1 bell pepper, sliced
6. 1 zucchini, sliced
7. 1 can coconut milk
8. 2 tablespoons red curry paste
9. 1 tablespoon soy sauce
10. 1 tablespoon brown sugar
11. Salt and pepper to taste

- Instructions:
  1. Heat olive oil in a large skillet over medium heat.
  2. Add diced onion and minced garlic to the skillet, and sauté until softened and fragrant.
  3. Add chicken pieces to the skillet and cook until browned on all sides.
  4. Stir in sliced bell pepper and zucchini, and cook

until vegetables are tender-crisp.

5. In a small bowl, whisk together coconut milk, red curry paste, soy sauce, and brown sugar.
6. Pour the coconut curry mixture into the skillet with the chicken and vegetables. Stir well to combine.
7. Let simmer for 10-15 minutes, or until the chicken is cooked through and the sauce has thickened slightly.
8. Season with salt and pepper to taste.
9. Serve hot over cooked rice.

Honey Mustard Glazed Chicken:

- Ingredients:
  1. 4 boneless, skinless chicken breasts

2. Salt and pepper to taste
3. 1/4 cup honey
4. 2 tablespoons Dijon mustard
5. 1 tablespoon olive oil
6. 2 cloves garlic, minced

- Instructions:
    1. Preheat oven to 375°F (190°C).
    2. Season chicken breasts with salt and pepper.
    3. In a small bowl, whisk together honey, Dijon mustard, and minced garlic.
    4. Heat olive oil in an oven-safe skillet over medium-high heat.
    5. Sear chicken breasts in the skillet for 2-3 minutes on each side until golden brown.

6. Brush honey mustard glaze over the chicken breasts.
7. Transfer the skillet to the preheated oven and bake for 20-25 minutes, or until chicken is cooked through.
8. Serve hot, garnished with fresh herbs if desired.

Grilled Lemon Herb Shrimp Skewers:

- Ingredients:
    1. 1 lb large shrimp, peeled and deveined
    2. Zest and juice of 1 lemon
    3. 2 tablespoons olive oil
    4. 2 cloves garlic, minced
    5. 1 tablespoon chopped fresh parsley
    6. 1 teaspoon dried oregano
    7. Salt and pepper to taste
    8. Skewers, soaked in water if wooden
- Instructions:

1. In a bowl, combine shrimp, lemon zest, lemon juice, olive oil, minced garlic, chopped parsley, dried oregano, salt, and pepper. Toss to coat the shrimp evenly.
2. Thread shrimp onto skewers.
3. Preheat grill to medium-high heat.
4. Grill shrimp skewers for 2-3 minutes per side, or until shrimp are pink and opaque.
5. Remove from grill and serve hot.

Turkey Meatball Soup:

- Ingredients:
    1. 1 lb ground turkey
    2. 1/4 cup breadcrumbs
    3. 1 egg
    4. 2 cloves garlic, minced

5. 1 onion, diced
6. 2 carrots, diced
7. 2 celery stalks, diced
8. 6 cups chicken broth
9. 1 can diced tomatoes
10. 1 teaspoon dried oregano
11. 1 teaspoon dried thyme
12. Salt and pepper to taste

- Instructions:
    1. In a bowl, combine ground turkey, breadcrumbs, egg, minced garlic, salt, and pepper. Mix until well combined, then shape into meatballs.
    2. In a large pot, heat olive oil over medium heat. Add diced onion, carrots, and celery, and cook until softened.
    3. Stir in dried oregano and dried thyme.

4. Add chicken broth and diced tomatoes to the pot. Bring to a simmer.
5. Gently drop turkey meatballs into the simmering broth.
6. Let soup simmer for 15-20 minutes, or until meatballs are cooked through and vegetables are tender.
7. Season with additional salt and pepper if needed.
8. Serve hot, optionally garnished with chopped parsley.

Lemon Garlic Butter Salmon:

- Ingredients:
    1. 4 salmon fillets
    2. Salt and pepper to taste
    3. 2 tablespoons olive oil
    4. 4 tablespoons unsalted butter
    5. 4 cloves garlic, minced

6. Zest and juice of 1 lemon

7. 2 tablespoons chopped fresh parsley

- Instructions:

1. Season salmon fillets with salt and pepper.

2. In a skillet, heat olive oil over medium heat.

3. Add salmon fillets to the skillet and cook for 4-5 minutes per side, or until salmon is cooked through and flakes easily with a fork. Remove from skillet and set aside.

4. In the same skillet, melt butter over medium heat. Add minced garlic and cook until fragrant.

5. Stir in lemon zest and lemon juice, then return cooked salmon fillets to the skillet.

6. Spoon lemon garlic butter sauce over the salmon fillets.
7. Sprinkle chopped parsley over the salmon.
8. Serve hot.

Chicken and Vegetable Stir-Fry with Cashews:

- Ingredients:
    1. 1 lb boneless, skinless chicken breasts, cut into thin strips
    2. Salt and pepper to taste
    3. 2 tablespoons soy sauce
    4. 1 tablespoon sesame oil
    5. 2 tablespoons olive oil
    6. 2 cloves garlic, minced
    7. 1 onion, sliced
    8. 2 cups mixed vegetables (such as bell peppers, broccoli, snow peas)
    9. 1/2 cup unsalted cashews
- Instructions:

1. Season chicken strips with salt, pepper, and soy sauce. Let marinate for 15-20 minutes.
2. Heat sesame oil and olive oil in a large skillet or wok over medium-high heat.
3. Add minced garlic and sliced onion to the skillet, and cook until softened and fragrant.
4. Add marinated chicken strips to the skillet and stir-fry until cooked through.
5. Add mixed vegetables to the skillet and continue stir-frying until vegetables are tender-crisp.
6. Stir in unsalted cashews and cook for an additional minute.
7. Serve hot over cooked rice or noodles.

Beef Stew:

- Ingredients:
    1. 1 lb stew beef, cut into bite-sized pieces
    2. 2 tablespoons olive oil
    3. 1 onion, diced
    4. 2 cloves garlic, minced
    5. 2 carrots, peeled and diced
    6. 2 celery stalks, diced
    7. 2 potatoes, peeled and diced
    8. 4 cups beef broth
    9. 1 can diced tomatoes
    10. 1 teaspoon dried thyme
    11. 1 teaspoon dried rosemary
    12. Salt and pepper to taste
- Instructions:
    1. Heat olive oil in a large pot over medium heat.

2. Add diced onion and minced garlic to the pot, and sauté until softened and fragrant.
3. Add stew beef to the pot and cook until browned on all sides.
4. Stir in diced carrots, celery, and potatoes.
5. Pour beef broth and diced tomatoes into the pot. Season with dried thyme, dried rosemary, salt, and pepper.
6. Bring stew to a simmer, then reduce heat to low and cover. Let simmer for 1-2 hours, stirring occasionally, until beef and vegetables are tender.
7. Adjust seasoning if needed.

8. Serve hot, optionally garnished with chopped parsley.

Baked Meatballs in Marinara Sauce:

- Ingredients:
    1. 1 lb ground beef
    2. 1/2 cup breadcrumbs
    3. 1/4 cup grated Parmesan cheese
    4. 1 egg
    5. 2 cloves garlic, minced
    6. 2 cups marinara sauce
    7. Salt and pepper to taste
- Instructions:
    1. Preheat oven to 375°F (190°C).
    2. In a bowl, combine ground beef, breadcrumbs, grated Parmesan cheese, egg, minced garlic, salt, and pepper. Mix until well combined.

3. Shape the mixture into meatballs and place them on a baking sheet lined with parchment paper.
4. Bake meatballs in the preheated oven for 20-25 minutes, or until cooked through and browned.
5. In a saucepan, heat marinara sauce over medium heat.
6. Add baked meatballs to the marinara sauce and let simmer for 10-15 minutes.
7. Serve hot, optionally garnished with additional grated Parmesan cheese and chopped parsley.

Steak with Mushroom Sauce:

- Ingredients:
    1. 4 beef steaks (such as sirloin or ribeye)
    2. Salt and pepper to taste

3. 2 tablespoons olive oil
4. 2 tablespoons unsalted butter
5. 2 cups sliced mushrooms
6. 2 cloves garlic, minced
7. 1/2 cup beef broth
8. 1/4 cup heavy cream
9. 1 tablespoon chopped fresh parsley

- Instructions:
    1. Season beef steaks with salt and pepper.
    2. Heat olive oil in a skillet over medium-high heat.
    3. Add beef steaks to the skillet and cook to desired doneness, about 4-5 minutes per side for medium-rare.
    4. Remove steaks from the skillet and let rest.
    5. In the same skillet, melt unsalted butter over medium heat. Add sliced

mushrooms and minced garlic, and cook until mushrooms are golden brown and tender.

6. Pour beef broth into the skillet and stir to deglaze the pan.
7. Stir in heavy cream and chopped parsley, and let simmer for a few minutes until sauce thickens slightly.
8. Serve cooked steaks topped with mushroom sauce.

Slow Cooker Pot Roast:

- Ingredients:
    1. 3-4 lbs beef chuck roast
    2. Salt and pepper to taste
    3. 2 tablespoons olive oil
    4. 1 onion, sliced
    5. 4 carrots, peeled and chopped

6. 4 celery stalks, chopped
7. 4 cloves garlic, minced
8. 2 cups beef broth
9. 1 tablespoon Worcestershire sauce
10. 2 bay leaves

- Instructions:
    1. Season beef chuck roast with salt and pepper.
    2. Heat olive oil in a large skillet over medium-high heat.
    3. Sear the beef chuck roast in the skillet until browned on all sides.
    4. Transfer the seared roast to a slow cooker.
    5. Add sliced onion, chopped carrots, chopped celery, minced garlic, beef broth, Worcestershire sauce, and bay leaves to the slow cooker.

6. Cover and cook on low heat for 8 hours or on high heat for 4-5 hours, until beef is tender and falling apart.
7. Remove bay leaves before serving.
8. Serve hot, with vegetables and juices from the slow cooker.

Spaghetti Bolognese:

- Ingredients:
    1. 8 oz spaghetti
    2. 1 lb ground beef
    3. 1 onion, diced
    4. 2 cloves garlic, minced
    5. 1 carrot, grated
    6. 1 celery stalk, diced
    7. 1 can diced tomatoes
    8. 1/2 cup beef broth
    9. 2 tablespoons tomato paste

10. 1 teaspoon dried oregano

11. Salt and pepper to taste

12. Grated Parmesan cheese for serving

- Instructions:
    1. Cook spaghetti according to package instructions. Drain and set aside.
    2. In a large skillet, brown ground beef over medium heat, breaking it apart with a spoon as it cooks.
    3. Add diced onion, minced garlic, grated carrot, and diced celery to the skillet. Cook until vegetables are softened.
    4. Stir in diced tomatoes, beef broth, tomato paste, dried oregano, salt, and pepper.
    5. Let the sauce simmer for 15-20 minutes, stirring

occasionally, until flavors are well combined and sauce has thickened slightly.

6. Serve cooked spaghetti topped with Bolognese sauce.

7. Sprinkle grated Parmesan cheese over the pasta before serving.

Beef and Vegetable Stir-Fry:

- Ingredients:
  1. 1 lb beef sirloin, thinly sliced
  2. 2 tablespoons soy sauce
  3. 1 tablespoon cornstarch
  4. 2 tablespoons olive oil
  5. 2 cloves garlic, minced
  6. 1 onion, sliced
  7. 2 bell peppers, sliced
  8. 2 cups broccoli florets
  9. 1 cup snap peas

10. Cooked rice or noodles, for serving

- Instructions:
    1. In a bowl, mix together soy sauce and cornstarch. Add sliced beef and toss to coat. Let marinate for 15-20 minutes.
    2. Heat olive oil in a large skillet or wok over medium-high heat.
    3. Add minced garlic and sliced onion to the skillet, and cook until softened.
    4. Add marinated beef to the skillet and stir-fry until browned.
    5. Add sliced bell peppers, broccoli florets, and snap peas to the skillet. Stir-fry until vegetables are tender-crisp.
    6. Serve hot over cooked rice or noodles.

Beef and Barley Soup:

- Ingredients:
    1. 1 lb stew beef, cut into bite-sized pieces
    2. Salt and pepper to taste
    3. 2 tablespoons olive oil
    4. 1 onion, diced
    5. 2 carrots, diced
    6. 2 celery stalks, diced
    7. 2 cloves garlic, minced
    8. 1 cup pearl barley
    9. 6 cups beef broth
    10. 1 teaspoon dried thyme
    11. 1 teaspoon dried rosemary
- Instructions:
    1. Season stew beef with salt and pepper.
    2. Heat olive oil in a large pot over medium heat.
    3. Add diced onion, carrots, celery, and minced garlic to the pot. Cook until softened.

4. Add seasoned stew beef to the pot and cook until browned on all sides.

5. Stir in pearl barley, beef broth, dried thyme, and dried rosemary.

6. Bring soup to a simmer, then reduce heat to low and cover. Let simmer for 1-2 hours, stirring occasionally, until beef is tender and barley is cooked.

7. Adjust seasoning if needed.

8. Serve hot, optionally garnished with chopped parsley.

Beef and Broccoli Stir-Fry:

- Ingredients:
  1. 1 lb flank steak, thinly sliced
  2. 1/4 cup soy sauce

3. 2 tablespoons brown sugar
4. 2 cloves garlic, minced
5. 1 teaspoon grated fresh ginger
6. 2 tablespoons olive oil
7. 2 cups broccoli florets
8. Cooked rice, for serving

- Instructions:
  1. In a bowl, whisk together soy sauce, brown sugar, minced garlic, and grated ginger. Add sliced flank steak and toss to coat. Let marinate for 15-20 minutes.
  2. Heat olive oil in a large skillet or wok over medium-high heat.
  3. Add marinated flank steak to the skillet and stir-fry until browned.
  4. Add broccoli florets to the skillet and stir-fry until tender-crisp.

5. Serve hot over cooked rice.

Beef Shepherd's Pie:

- Ingredients:
    1. 1 lb ground beef
    2. 1 onion, diced
    3. 2 carrots, diced
    4. 2 cloves garlic, minced
    5. 1 cup frozen peas
    6. 1 cup beef broth
    7. 2 tablespoons tomato paste
    8. 2 tablespoons Worcestershire sauce
    9. 4 cups mashed potatoes
    10. Salt and pepper to taste
    11. Chopped fresh parsley for garnish
- Instructions:
    1. Preheat oven to 375°F (190°C).
    2. In a skillet, brown ground beef over medium heat. Drain excess fat.

3. Add diced onion, carrots, and minced garlic to the skillet. Cook until vegetables are softened.

4. Stir in frozen peas, beef broth, tomato paste, and Worcestershire sauce. Simmer for 10-15 minutes until flavors are well combined and sauce has thickened slightly.

5. Season with salt and pepper to taste.

6. Transfer the beef mixture to a baking dish.

7. Spread mashed potatoes evenly over the beef mixture.

8. Bake in the preheated oven for 25-30 minutes, or until the top is golden brown.

9. Garnish with chopped fresh parsley before serving.

Beef Chili:

- Ingredients:
    1. 1 lb ground beef
    2. 1 onion, diced
    3. 2 cloves garlic, minced
    4. 1 bell pepper, diced
    5. 1 can kidney beans, drained and rinsed
    6. 1 can diced tomatoes
    7. 1 cup beef broth
    8. 2 tablespoons chili powder
    9. 1 teaspoon ground cumin
    10. Salt and pepper to taste
    11. Olive oil for cooking
- Instructions:
    1. Heat olive oil in a large pot over medium heat.
    2. Add diced onion, minced garlic, and diced bell

pepper to the pot. Cook until softened.

3. Add ground beef to the pot and cook until browned, breaking it apart with a spoon as it cooks.

4. Stir in kidney beans, diced tomatoes, beef broth, chili powder, ground cumin, salt, and pepper.

5. Bring chili to a simmer, then reduce heat to low and cover. Let simmer for 30-40 minutes, stirring occasionally.

6. Adjust seasoning if needed.

7. Serve hot, optionally garnished with shredded cheese, sour cream, or chopped green onions.

Banana Oatmeal Cookies:

- Ingredients:
    1. 2 ripe bananas, mashed
    2. 1 cup rolled oats
    3. 1/4 cup chopped nuts (such as walnuts or pecans) (optional)
    4. 1/4 cup raisins or dried cranberries (optional)
    5. 1 teaspoon cinnamon
- Instructions:
    1. Preheat oven to 350°F (175°C) and line a baking sheet with parchment paper.
    2. In a bowl, combine mashed bananas, rolled oats, chopped nuts, raisins or dried cranberries (if using), and cinnamon. Mix well.

3. Drop spoonfuls of the mixture onto the prepared baking sheet, spacing them apart.
4. Flatten each cookie slightly with the back of a spoon.
5. Bake in the preheated oven for 12-15 minutes, or until cookies are golden brown and set.
6. Allow cookies to cool on the baking sheet for a few minutes before transferring to a wire rack to cool completely.
7. Enjoy these naturally sweetened cookies as a healthier dessert option.

Yogurt Parfait:

- Ingredients:
  1. 1 cup Greek yogurt
  2. 1 tablespoon honey or maple syrup

3. 1/4 cup granola
4. 1/2 cup mixed berries (such as strawberries, blueberries, raspberries)
5. 1 tablespoon chopped nuts (such as almonds or walnuts) (optional)

- Instructions:
    1. In a glass or bowl, layer Greek yogurt, honey or maple syrup, granola, mixed berries, and chopped nuts (if using).
    2. Repeat the layers until the glass or bowl is filled.
    3. Serve immediately as a refreshing and nutritious dessert option.

Baked Apples with Cinnamon and Walnuts:

- Ingredients:
    1. 4 apples (such as Granny Smith or Honeycrisp)

2. 1/4 cup chopped walnuts
3. 2 tablespoons honey or maple syrup
4. 1 teaspoon cinnamon
5. 1/4 cup water

- Instructions:
    1. Preheat oven to 375°F (190°C).
    2. Core each apple and remove the seeds, creating a well in the center.
    3. In a bowl, mix together chopped walnuts, honey or maple syrup, and cinnamon.
    4. Stuff each cored apple with the walnut mixture.
    5. Place stuffed apples in a baking dish and pour water into the bottom of the dish.
    6. Cover the baking dish with foil and bake in the preheated oven for 30-35

minutes, or until apples are tender.

7. Serve baked apples warm, optionally topped with a dollop of Greek yogurt or a drizzle of additional honey or maple syrup.

Chocolate Avocado Mousse:

- Ingredients:
  1. 2 ripe avocados
  2. 1/4 cup cocoa powder
  3. 1/4 cup honey or maple syrup
  4. 1 teaspoon vanilla extract
  5. Pinch of salt
- Instructions:
  1. Scoop the flesh of the avocados into a blender or food processor.
  2. Add cocoa powder, honey or maple syrup, vanilla extract, and a pinch of salt.

3. Blend until smooth and creamy, scraping down the sides of the blender or food processor as needed.
4. Transfer the chocolate avocado mousse to serving dishes.
5. Chill in the refrigerator for at least 30 minutes before serving.
6. Enjoy this rich and indulgent dessert with a healthier twist.

Fruit Salad with Honey-Lime Dressing:

- Ingredients:
    1. 2 cups mixed fruit (such as strawberries, grapes, pineapple, kiwi, oranges)
    2. 1 tablespoon honey
    3. Juice of 1 lime
    4. Fresh mint leaves for garnish (optional)
- Instructions:

1. Wash and prepare the mixed fruit as needed, cutting larger fruits into bite-sized pieces.
2. In a small bowl, whisk together honey and lime juice to make the dressing.
3. Drizzle the honey-lime dressing over the mixed fruit and toss gently to coat.
4. Garnish with fresh mint leaves if desired.
5. Serve the fruit salad immediately as a refreshing and naturally sweet dessert option.

Chapter 15:NUTRIENT BOOSTING RECIPES

Spinach and Berry Smoothie:
- Ingredients:

1. 2 cups fresh spinach leaves
2. 1 cup mixed berries (such as strawberries, blueberries, raspberries)
3. 1 ripe banana
4. 1/2 cup Greek yogurt
5. 1 tablespoon honey or maple syrup (optional)
6. 1 cup almond milk or any milk of choice

- Instructions:
    1. Place spinach leaves, mixed berries, banana, Greek yogurt, honey or maple syrup (if using), and almond milk in a blender.
    2. Blend until smooth and creamy.
    3. Pour the smoothie into glasses and serve immediately as a nutrient-packed breakfast or snack.

Quinoa Salad with Chickpeas and Vegetables:

- o Ingredients:
    1. 1 cup quinoa, rinsed
    2. 2 cups water or vegetable broth
    3. 1 can chickpeas, drained and rinsed
    4. 1 cucumber, diced
    5. 1 bell pepper, diced
    6. 1/4 cup chopped fresh parsley
    7. Juice of 1 lemon
    8. 2 tablespoons olive oil
    9. Salt and pepper to taste
- o Instructions:
    1. In a medium saucepan, bring water or vegetable broth to a boil. Add quinoa, reduce heat to low, cover, and simmer for 15-20 minutes, or until quinoa is cooked and

water is absorbed. Remove from heat and let cool.

2. In a large bowl, combine cooked quinoa, chickpeas, diced cucumber, diced bell pepper, and chopped fresh parsley.

3. In a small bowl, whisk together lemon juice, olive oil, salt, and pepper to make the dressing.

4. Pour the dressing over the quinoa salad and toss gently to combine.

5. Serve chilled or at room temperature as a nutrient-rich lunch or side dish.

Salmon and Asparagus Foil Packets:

- Ingredients:
  1. 4 salmon fillets
  2. 1 bunch asparagus, trimmed

3. 2 tablespoons olive oil
        4. 2 cloves garlic, minced
        5. Zest and juice of 1 lemon
        6. Salt and pepper to taste
   ○ Instructions:
        1. Preheat oven to 375°F (190°C).
        2. Cut four large pieces of aluminum foil.
        3. Place a salmon fillet on each piece of foil.
        4. Arrange asparagus spears around each salmon fillet.
        5. In a small bowl, whisk together olive oil, minced garlic, lemon zest, lemon juice, salt, and pepper.
        6. Drizzle the olive oil mixture over the salmon and asparagus in each foil packet.
        7. Fold the edges of the foil over the salmon and

asparagus to create sealed packets.

8. Place the foil packets on a baking sheet and bake in the preheated oven for 15-20 minutes, or until salmon is cooked through and asparagus is tender.
9. Carefully open the foil packets and serve hot.

Turkey and Vegetable Stir-Fry:

- Ingredients:
    1. 1 lb ground turkey
    2. 2 tablespoons olive oil
    3. 2 cloves garlic, minced
    4. 1 onion, sliced
    5. 2 carrots, julienned
    6. 2 bell peppers, sliced
    7. 2 cups broccoli florets
    8. 1/4 cup soy sauce
    9. 1 tablespoon honey or maple syrup

10. Cooked brown rice, for serving

○ Instructions:

1. Heat olive oil in a large skillet or wok over medium-high heat.

2. Add minced garlic and sliced onion to the skillet, and cook until softened and fragrant.

3. Add ground turkey to the skillet and cook until browned, breaking it apart with a spoon as it cooks.

4. Stir in julienned carrots, sliced bell peppers, and broccoli florets. Cook until vegetables are tender-crisp.

5. In a small bowl, whisk together soy sauce and honey or maple syrup. Pour over the turkey and

vegetable mixture in the skillet.

6. Stir well to combine and let simmer for a few minutes.
7. Serve hot over cooked brown rice.

Greek Yogurt Berry Parfait:

- Ingredients:
    1. 2 cups Greek yogurt
    2. 1 cup mixed berries (such as strawberries, blueberries, raspberries)
    3. 1/4 cup granola
    4. 1 tablespoon honey or maple syrup
- Instructions:
    1. In serving glasses or bowls, layer Greek yogurt, mixed berries, granola, and honey or maple syrup.
    2. Repeat the layers until glasses or bowls are filled.

3. Serve immediately as a nutritious and satisfying dessert or snack option.

Quinoa Salad with Roasted Vegetables:

- Ingredients:
    1. 1 cup quinoa, rinsed
    2. 2 cups water or vegetable broth
    3. 2 cups mixed vegetables (such as bell peppers, zucchini, cherry tomatoes)
    4. 2 tablespoons olive oil
    5. 2 cloves garlic, minced
    6. Juice of 1 lemon
    7. Salt and pepper to taste
    8. Fresh herbs (such as parsley or basil), chopped (optional)
- Instructions:
    1. Preheat oven to 400°F (200°C).

2. In a saucepan, bring water or vegetable broth to a boil. Add quinoa, reduce heat to low, cover, and simmer for 15-20 minutes, or until quinoa is cooked and liquid is absorbed. Remove from heat and let cool.

3. Meanwhile, spread mixed vegetables on a baking sheet. Drizzle with olive oil, minced garlic, salt, and pepper, and toss to coat.

4. Roast vegetables in the preheated oven for 20-25 minutes, or until tender and slightly caramelized.

5. In a large bowl, combine cooked quinoa and roasted vegetables. Squeeze lemon juice over the mixture and toss to combine.

6. Season with additional salt and pepper if needed.
7. Garnish with chopped fresh herbs if desired.
8. Serve warm or at room temperature as a nutritious and satisfying meal.

Stuffed Bell Peppers with Turkey and Quinoa:

- Ingredients:
  1. 4 large bell peppers, halved and seeds removed
  2. 1 cup quinoa, cooked
  3. 1 lb ground turkey
  4. 1 onion, diced
  5. 2 cloves garlic, minced
  6. 1 can diced tomatoes
  7. 1 teaspoon dried oregano
  8. 1 teaspoon dried basil
  9. Salt and pepper to taste

10. 1/2 cup shredded cheese (such as mozzarella or cheddar) (optional)

- Instructions:
  1. Preheat oven to 375°F (190°C).
  2. In a skillet, cook ground turkey over medium heat until browned. Add diced onion and minced garlic, and cook until softened.
  3. Stir in cooked quinoa, diced tomatoes, dried oregano, dried basil, salt, and pepper. Cook for an additional 5 minutes.
  4. Arrange bell pepper halves in a baking dish.
  5. Spoon the turkey and quinoa mixture into each bell pepper half.
  6. If using, sprinkle shredded cheese over the stuffed peppers.

7. Cover the baking dish with foil and bake in the preheated oven for 25-30 minutes, or until peppers are tender.
8. Remove foil and bake for an additional 5 minutes to melt the cheese (if using).
9. Serve hot as a healthy and filling meal option.

Baked Salmon with Lemon and Dill:

- Ingredients:
    1. 4 salmon fillets
    2. Salt and pepper to taste
    3. 2 tablespoons olive oil
    4. Zest and juice of 1 lemon
    5. 2 tablespoons chopped fresh dill
    6. Lemon slices for garnish (optional)
- Instructions:
    1. Preheat oven to 375°F (190°C).

2. Season salmon fillets with salt and pepper.

3. In a small bowl, whisk together olive oil, lemon zest, lemon juice, and chopped fresh dill.

4. Place salmon fillets on a baking sheet lined with parchment paper.

5. Drizzle the lemon and dill mixture over the salmon fillets.

6. If desired, place lemon slices on top of each salmon fillet for additional flavor.

7. Bake in the preheated oven for 12-15 minutes, or until salmon is cooked through and flakes easily with a fork.

8. Serve hot with your choice of side dishes, such as

roasted vegetables or quinoa salad.

Turkey and Vegetable Soup:

- Ingredients:
    1. 1 lb ground turkey
    2. 1 onion, diced
    3. 2 carrots, diced
    4. 2 celery stalks, diced
    5. 2 cloves garlic, minced
    6. 6 cups chicken broth
    7. 1 can diced tomatoes
    8. 1 cup quinoa, rinsed
    9. 1 teaspoon dried thyme
    10. Salt and pepper to taste
    11. Fresh parsley for garnish (optional)
- Instructions:
    1. In a large pot, cook ground turkey over medium heat until browned. Add diced onion, carrots, celery, and minced garlic, and cook

until vegetables are softened.

2. Stir in chicken broth, diced tomatoes, rinsed quinoa, dried thyme, salt, and pepper.

3. Bring soup to a simmer, then reduce heat to low and cover. Let simmer for 15-20 minutes, or until quinoa is cooked and vegetables are tender.

4. Adjust seasoning if needed.

5. Serve hot, optionally garnished with chopped fresh parsley for extra flavor.

Grilled Chicken Salad with Balsamic Vinaigrette:

- Ingredients:
  1. 2 boneless, skinless chicken breasts

2. Salt and pepper to taste
3. 6 cups mixed salad greens
4. 1 cup cherry tomatoes, halved
5. 1 cucumber, sliced
6. 1/4 cup sliced red onion
7. 1/4 cup crumbled feta cheese
8. 2 tablespoons chopped fresh basil
9. 2 tablespoons balsamic vinegar
10. 1 tablespoon olive oil

- Instructions:

1. Preheat grill to medium-high heat.
2. Season chicken breasts with salt and pepper.
3. Grill chicken breasts for 6-8 minutes per side, or until cooked through and no longer pink in the center.

4. Remove chicken from grill and let rest for a few minutes before slicing.
5. In a large bowl, combine mixed salad greens, cherry tomatoes, sliced cucumber, sliced red onion, crumbled feta cheese, and chopped fresh basil.
6. In a small bowl, whisk together balsamic vinegar and olive oil to make the vinaigrette.
7. Add sliced grilled chicken to the salad, and drizzle with balsamic vinaigrette.
8. Toss gently to combine.
9. Serve immediately as a light and refreshing meal option.

Vegetable Hummus Platter:

- Ingredients:
    1. 1 cup hummus
    2. Assorted raw vegetables (such as carrots, cucumber, bell peppers, cherry tomatoes)
    3. Whole grain crackers or pita bread
- Instructions:
    1. Arrange the hummus in the center of a serving platter.
    2. Surround the hummus with assorted raw vegetables and whole grain crackers or pita bread.
    3. Serve as a nutritious and satisfying appetizer or snack option.

Baked Sweet Potato Fries:

- Ingredients:
    1. 2 medium sweet potatoes, peeled and cut into fries
    2. 2 tablespoons olive oil
    3. 1 teaspoon paprika
    4. 1/2 teaspoon garlic powder
    5. Salt and pepper to taste
- Instructions:
    1. Preheat oven to 425°F (220°C) and line a baking sheet with parchment paper.
    2. In a large bowl, toss sweet potato fries with olive oil, paprika, garlic powder, salt, and pepper until evenly coated.
    3. Spread sweet potato fries in a single layer on the prepared baking sheet.
    4. Bake in the preheated oven for 20-25 minutes, flipping halfway through,

until fries are golden
brown and crispy.

5. Serve hot as a delicious
   and nutritious snack
   option.

Caprese Skewers:

- Ingredients:
  1. Cherry tomatoes
  2. Fresh mozzarella balls
     (bocconcini)
  3. Fresh basil leaves
  4. Balsamic glaze
     (store-bought or
     homemade)
  5. Toothpicks or small
     skewers
- Instructions:
  1. Thread one cherry tomato,
     one mozzarella ball, and
     one basil leaf onto each
     toothpick or skewer.

2. Arrange the caprese skewers on a serving platter.
3. Drizzle with balsamic glaze just before serving.
4. Serve as a light and refreshing appetizer option.

Greek Yogurt Dip with Veggie Sticks:

- Ingredients:
    1. 1 cup Greek yogurt
    2. 1 tablespoon lemon juice
    3. 1 clove garlic, minced
    4. 1 tablespoon chopped fresh dill (or 1 teaspoon dried dill)
    5. Salt and pepper to taste
    6. Assorted raw vegetable sticks (such as carrots, celery, bell peppers)
- Instructions:
    1. In a bowl, mix together Greek yogurt, lemon juice,

minced garlic, chopped fresh dill, salt, and pepper until well combined.
2. Transfer the yogurt dip to a serving bowl.
3. Arrange assorted raw vegetable sticks around the yogurt dip.
4. Serve chilled as a healthy and flavorful snack option.

Stuffed Dates with Almonds and Goat Cheese:

- o Ingredients:
    1. Medjool dates, pitted
    2. Whole almonds
    3. Goat cheese
- o Instructions:
    1. Slice each date lengthwise and remove the pit.
    2. Fill each date with a whole almond and a small amount of goat cheese.

3. Press the date halves together to enclose the filling.
4. Arrange the stuffed dates on a serving platter.
5. Serve as a sweet and savory appetizer or snack option.

CONCLUSION

"Congratulations on completing the 30-Minute Solution Parkinson's Diet Cookbook for Seniors! You've taken a crucial step towards managing your Parkinson's disease and improving your overall health and well-being.

Remember, cooking and nutrition don't have to be overwhelming or time-consuming. With the simple and delicious recipes in this cookbook, you can enjoy healthy and balanced meals in just 30 minutes or less.

Don't let Parkinson's disease hold you back - take control of your diet and nutrition today! With the 30-Minute Solution Parkinson's Diet Cookbook for Seniors, you have the tools and confidence to:

- Manage your symptoms and slow disease progression
- Improve your overall health and well-being
- Enjoy delicious and nutritious meals with ease
- Take charge of your cooking and nutrition

Keep cooking, keep smiling, and remember to always prioritize your health and happiness!

Bonus: Share your favorite recipes with loved ones and start cooking together - it's a great way to stay connected and supported on your Parkinson's journey!"

This conclusion aims to:

- Congratulate the reader on completing the cookbook
- Emphasize the importance of taking control of diet and nutrition
- Encourage the reader to continue cooking and prioritizing their health
- Offer a final motivational boost
- End with a positive and uplifting note

THE END